WISHES WON'T WASH DISHES!

A guide to turn your health wishes into reality

Sheri Fisher, Ph.D.

Author of *A New Hope for Health* books including the
<u>I Love to Eat!</u> cookbook series

Published by
A New Hope for Health

Graphic Artist
Ralph Huddlestone

Design and layout
HSA
4 West 43rd Street
New York, NY 10036

International Standard Book Number (ISBN): 0-9726037-0-0

Printed in the United States of America
1st Printing

Order copies from:

A New Hope for Health
P.O. Box 654
St. George, UT 84770

website: anewhopeforhealth.com
email: anewhopeforhealth@infowest.com

ACKNOWLEDGEMENTS

Many people have been instrumental in the development of this. A special thanks to my husband, Brian, for his help and support in the technical aspect of compiling this book, and also his insights from everyday experiences in our Southern Utah based health business. – A New Hope for Health.

Especially to my sons, Cameron and Royce, who patiently grew up with mom taking classes and trying out her new education and ideas to help encourage a healthy lifestyle. Although based on religious beliefs and study, a healthy diet, exercise, and the importance of abstaining from harmful substances were a training priority throughout their childhood years.

Thanks to Dawn Rotert who spent valuable time proofreading for clarity and grammar. Also to Hart Wixom, editor, who helped me to get this book ready for publishing.

I appreciate Ralph Huddestone (my step-dad) for all of the time, expertise, and creativity in the design of the cover and layout of this book. Thanks goes to my mom, Donna, for her wise insight in identifying some of the barriers to ultimate health and helping with the evolution of the title.

A special thanks to all who have asked questions about health and encouraging my continued studies and research.

NOTICE TO READERS

DEDICATION

I dedicate this work to my family, in hopes that some or all of this information may be beneficial to their health and well being. And, to anyone who wishes to improve his/her life by being the their best and healthiest self.

CONTENTS

INTRODUCTION

When I ask people why they became interested in health or why they are working in the health field, they usually have a story to tell. My story began about 23 years ago. My first son was only 2 years old when the doctor informed me that I should consider having his tonsils removed. He had been sick most of the winter and each time I took him into the doctor, it was the same diagnosis-tonsillitis. The doctor recommended that I have his tonsils removed. This and other common illnesses seemed to becoming a way of life for us and it was miserable for all. No matter how much I "wished" him better, it just wasn't happening! I decided then that "wishes won't wash dishes!" In other words, I was going to do something. I would have to take responsibility for our health and see if I could figure out what *I* could *do* to help my son avoid a tonsillectomy.

I began studying and reading everything I could find. That many years ago there was not as much information out on nutrition and health as there is now. But, what I did discover was that dairy products, with their mucous forming properties, had been known to cause many childhood illnesses such as tonsillitis, bronchitis, ear infections, bed-wetting, asthma, childhood onset diabetes, etc. I immediately took him off dairy products and to this day he has not had one more episode of tonsillitis and of course still has his tonsils. I was amazed that diet and nutrition could have such an impact on our health. I realized that our health is something we do have much control over. Not only nutrition but there are other areas that can impact our life.

This manual was written as a guideline for anyone wishing to improve their health, lose weight, gain more energy and vitality, reduce stress, or improve the environment and the ecology of our planet. It has been written in a workbook form so the reader may work through the chapters and arrive at their own solutions to various issues where needed. Each chapter can be used independently or together depending upon the concerns of the reader.

It is not an in depth technical book, but it is written so that the average person can understand the basic information and reasoning behind the recommendations. Recommended reading is listed at the end of the book for more detailed information. If the guidelines are followed, the information provided in this manual can enhance mental, emotional, physical, and spiritual health, and well being.

Fortunately, our health is one area we do have much control over. We must take responsibility for our own well being and not turn it over to others to fix, or solve our problems. There are many health problems we can improve on or solve on our own. It is a wonderful feeling to be in control of our lives, our desires, our thoughts, our actions, our health and most importantly – our decisions. There are many health problems that must be cared for by a competent healthcare practitioner. But, even in these situations, there is still a lot we can do on our own to enhance and help the healing process along more quickly and efficiently.

This manual was not meant to offend, criticize, judge or condemn, but is offered as information and education to help us become a happier, healthier, energetic, and fun loving people. The reader must choose for his/herself the messages gleaned from this manual, and must make a consistent effort to apply the principles if positive results are to be expected.

A great quote to sum it all up is, "It is better to prepare and prevent than to repair and repent." So the bottom line is, "we can take time to be healthy or we will have to take the time to be sick". What's the underlying message? You got it! Wishing won't cut it. We have to act!

As a disclaimer, it is understood that there are some conditions that are out of our control such as the results from accidents, birth defects, genetic abnormalities, and some chronic diseases. But, most of the health conditions my husband and I see each day in our health business and in the public school setting where I spend the majority of my day, can be improved upon or eliminated by a change or modification in lifestyles.

As we start to make changes in our lifestyle, here are some things to consider:

When making a dietary or lifestyle change, some people experience some discomfort or symptoms. This is from the detoxification process. If you experience any of the following symptoms then rest more, slow down a little on your changes, and increase your water intake to help speed up detoxification

- General fatigue
- Pains and aches
- Fever, chills, coldness, cough
- Skin eruptions/body odor
- Temporary decrease in sexual desire
- Temporary cessation menstruation
- Mental irritability
- Restless dreams, minor hair loss
- Depression
- Lack of coordination
- Headaches
- Shakiness/nervousness/tension
- Mucous elimination through the elimination channels

It is suggested that you use this manual for your written responses or keep a small journal. Write down your responses to the questions. Be sure to record your symptoms and how you feel, your feelings about the topic, how you may accomplish your goals, resources available to help you, etc.

When we write down our goals we are more committed to completing them. You can also refer back to your responses and chart your progress while making changes or additions in your program as needed.

CHAPTER 1
IDENTIFY AND OVERCOME BARRIERS TO ULTIMATE HEALTH

ASK YOURSELF,
"HOW MUCH HEALTH DO I REALLY WANT?"

Would you believe that there are some people who do really do not want to get well? "No", you say? "Why would anyone not want to get well?"

If you are basically healthy or are presently working hard to improve your health, **then this chapter may not apply to you.** But, if you know of someone (possibly even yourself) who continuously goes to the doctor and either the doctor finds nothing wrong, or the person just never seems to get better, read on. *By identifying some of the barriers to optimal health and well being, you, or a loved one, may be on the road to recovery!*

As a counselor in the public school system and consultant to my husband in our health supportive business, we see many clients on a daily basis. We see health conditions ranging anywhere from structural problems, to fatigue, to digestive disturbances, to emotional or mental disorders, to chemical/hormonal imbalances, and to chronic health problems such as: heart disease, diabetes, and cancer. Who would not want to recover from or improve on any of these conditions? Surprisingly enough, either subconsciously or consciously, we have discovered that some people do not.

Can you think of some of the reasons why some people would not want to improve or eliminate their heath problems?

Through our interactions with friends, family and clients, we have also discovered some of the most common barriers why people feel they are "better off" being sick. Although generally negative in their outcome, I will refer to these barriers as "benefits".

Whether or not we realize it, we do things because we are receiving or perceiving some form of benefit. The benefits can end up being barriers to ultimate health. Benefits for staying sick usually have a negative impact on our life and/or others. But, as we will see, good health and a different perspective will be a more positive benefit in our life than any illness or condition could ever be. It is like fighting a losing battle to work so hard on improving your nutrition, your lifestyle, or your health if you are preventing good health by self-defeating behaviors or attitudes.

First, I will list many of the perceived "benefits" of remaining in a poor health condition. I will then explain the rationale behind them and give examples of how changing our perceptions of them will give us more positive benefits. As you read through these benefits, see if you (or someone you know) can identify with any of them.

BENEFITS FOR NOT
IMPROVING OUR HEALTH

1. I don't have to go to work.
2. I don't have to face my responsibilities.
3. I receive more attention.
4. I receive help and resources.
5. I don't have to worry about failure because I'm not required to try.
6. I can justify my illness because of my unworthiness.

7. I like playing the role of the martyr.
8. I don't have to give up my lifestyle
9. I can just accept my fate.
10. I can escape from my reality.

RATIONALE OF BENEFITS AND NEW POSITIVE PERCEPTIONS

1. **"I don't have to go to work"**. Recently, a lady was diagnosed with carpal tunnel syndrome. Instead of looking for a job that could allow this condition time to heal, or seeking a way to re-educate herself in a different field, she has filed for disability insurance.

If your job is not rewarding, fun, interesting, and satisfying, then it may be time to make a change. Maybe for you, going to work seems worse than the illness or condition itself. Perhaps you know of someone who looks for ways to obtain disability insurance and allow the system or others to support them? How often, though, do you think the "disability" is justified?

Sometimes we feel there is no way to change our job situation, but with the right resources you **can**. If you are not sure what you would like to do or what jobs may be available for your specific health condition, go to your nearest college career center or Job Service and talk to someone there about career options, education, interest, aptitude and ability inventories. A job that fills our needs increases our self-esteem, helps us to feel productive, and gives us new focus and enthusiasm.

Remember, without good health, you cannot even pursue an enjoyable hobby much less reach your career goals. Start improving your health now while you are identifying your new educational and career options. You will then be more prepared to make changes when the opportunities arise.

1. *What is it about the current job that you dread? (i.e. personnel, pay, hours, location)*

2. *Why would you have to return to or stay in that particular job? (i.e. no other training, family responsibilities, afraid to make a change)*

3. *How could you re-educate or train yourself (if necessary) to find a more rewarding job? (i.e., college career center, vocational training program, night classes, distance learning)*

4. *What are some of your favorite hobbies, abilities, and interests? Could one of them bring you an income?*

6. *What is your passion in life? Could this become a career?*

7. *Make a list of your options and resources. (i.e., family support, community college, student loans)*

2. I don't have to face my responsibilities. A young man was feeling overwhelmed with all of the responsibilities he had. More and more often, he became sick. Of course, his responsibilities became further and further behind. This leads to even more frustration.

Each of us has different responsibilities and obligations such as: children, spouse, parents, job, community, and church. Some of us take on too many responsibilities all at once and we become overwhelmed with trying to meet so many obligations. Some responsibilities will only be required of us for a period of time while others may be a life long commitment. With some responsibilities we have no choice but to meet them, while others we must stop and re-evaluate them in regards to our priorities. People and relationships are a big priority for most. When we "get out" of ourselves and serve others and help to meet *their* needs, ours in turn will be met. Happiness and satisfaction comes from doing for others.

1. *List your responsibilities and obligations. Beside each one, write down if you feel this particular responsibility is causing you to feel frustrated or overwhelmed and why.*

2. *Is this responsibility only for a period of time? (i.e. in a few years your last child will be on his/her own or this is only a temporary job until I complete my training). If so, they are easier to deal with knowing that "this too shall pass."*

3. *Could any of these responsibilities be postponed or re-assigned to someone else? (i.e. a church, job or community position).*

4. *Could you receive help or resources to assist you with a particular responsibility? (i.e. If you are taking care of an ill or elderly family member, could other members of the family share in the responsibility, do you need to learn how to manage time better?)*

5. *List some positive ways you can relieve some of the burdens you may be feeling while still filling the responsibilities and obligations you have committed to.*

3. I receive more attention. A woman diagnosed with M.S, spent most of her time in a wheel chair. She used her illness to what she thought was her advantage. Her constant need for assistance and incessant whining kept her husband endlessly caring for her. In her mind, he would not leave her because of her illness and the obligation he felt toward her. This made her feel secure and safe. Well, it only worked for a short time. He soon left her for another woman.

This is like the small child who consistently gets into trouble. He is scolded or spanked and yet continues to repeat the same offenses. If he is feeling that he is not receiving attention by being good, then he learns that he will receive attention when he is being bad. You see, in his mind, any attention (even negative) is better than no attention. That is why positive reinforcements change behavior – whereas negative reinforcements do not.

It is no different with people and their health conditions. When we are ill, we usually receive more attention from family, community, or church members than when we are healthy. If we are not secure in our relationships, or we feel we are not receiving as much attention as we would like, we will find a way to get the attention one way or another. But, if we will look for ways to help others suddenly we do not need as much help.

1. Is *this the* **kind** *of attention you really want?(i.e. sympathy, pity, obligation)*

2. *Who or what do you want to receive more attention from?(i.e. spouse, children, community)*

3. *What could be a more positive approach to receiving attention)? (i.e. giving service to others, having a positive attitude, trying to do things independently)*

4. *If you do not receive more attention from others once your health improves, can you still be secure enough in yourself to meet your own needs and go on with your life?*

4. **I receive help and resources.** A middle-aged woman with five young children, continuously sought help with meals, cleaning, babysitting, and companionship. She began to wear out her resources. People stopped calling or coming over. She became bitter and resentful because she felt that no one cared.

The help or resources we receive while we are ill can come in many forms and from many areas. We can receive others time, money, food, shelter, and clothing. Whether from our family, community, or church members, other people must help to meet our needs. This can be a great hardship on others who also have responsibilities of their own.

Usually when we receive this kind of help, our self-esteem suffers. This in turn makes us feel even worse. We generally wish to be self-sufficient, and it is difficult to depend on others to take care of our needs we know we should be meeting ourselves. Therefore, please consider the following.

1. *Are you causing any unnecessary hardships on your family, church, or community?(i.e., their time, resources, or stress levels)*

2. *Could any of your needs be met on your own? (i.e., financial, family, personal help)*

3. *Would you want to feel obligated to meet the needs of others that are in the same situation that you are in? If not, then why?*

4. *What could you do to lessen the demands on the various resources that you are using? (i.e. work part time, fix meals, tend own children)*

5. How could you show gratitude and give back to those people or organizations that have helped or benefited you? (i.e., send thank you cards, offer to do something for them in return, spend time in service to others)

5. I don't have to worry about failure because I'm not required to try. One man told me that he would like to continue with her education but feels inadequate because he was a high school drop out. He feels intimidated with others who completed their public education.

Many people would like to attempt challenging opportunities in their life but they are afraid to take the risk. Sometimes we make excuses, when we are afraid to attempt a challenging feat for fear we may not succeed such as "I'm not smart enough" or "I don't have that talent". We often use our health problems as reasons why we can't or won't try. Have you heard any of these? "I'm just too sick", ""I just know I can't do it", or "If you had my problems you couldn't do it either".

Failures are only setbacks. They do not mean **we** are a failure. It is often easier to use an excuse than to take on a challenge and try.

1. What are some of the health problems you sometimes use as an excuse to avoid trying something difficult? (i.e. getting a job, meeting new people, attempting a new hobby or returning to an old one)?

2. What would be the worst thing that could happen if you did not succeed? (i.e. people would laugh or be disappointed, embarrassment, change plans)

3. Would that experience be so terrible that you could

not attempt it or something else again? If yes, then why?

4. *Would you consider the set back a " roadblock" or a "stepping stone"?(In other words would it be a learning experience and a chance to grow or would it be a reason to not try again?)*

5. *Is the health condition really so severe that you <u>could</u> <u>not</u> be successful in the area(s) you are avoiding? (i.e. physically impossible to get out of bed, or involved in a serious accident and are still in the healing process). If yes, give your self the needed time to get back on your feet.*

Ghandi once said "Strength does not come from physical (or mental) capacity; it comes from an indomitable will."

6. **I can justify my illness(es) because of my unworthiness.** A young lady explained that because of choices she made in the past that her current health condition is now punishment. She feels there is nothing she can do now to improve her health.

Some people feel that they do not deserve good health. Sometimes they feel guilt or remorse because of past experiences. There are those individuals who, for some reason, have mishaps. Whether an accident, illness, or a choice, sometimes they feel it is just "bad luck" or "karma". Some things are out of our control, whereas others are **not**. The truth is – we often make our own luck.

I don't believe that we are on this earth to sit idly by and become a victim. There is much we can do to improve our health. If we are holding on to negative issues from the past, we must do all we can to rectify the situation. Mend the relationships. Seek forgiveness. Make restitution where possible. Make good choices in regards to our health. Once we have done all that we can do, we **must** move on. Only by letting go can we begin to heal physically, emotionally, mentally, and spiritually.

1. *List the various health conditions you have dealt with. Cross off the ones that were* **totally** *beyond your control. (i.e., a birth defect, an accident, abuse). Let them go mentally and emotionally as you look for ways to overcome your limitations or improve your condition.*

2. *Next, make a list of the issues that you could have had or do now have some control over. (i.e., weight problem, anger, stress related problems, poor choice)*

3. *What could you have done differently to have avoided that particular problem (i.e., made a different choice, dealt with the stress or anger more appropriately, learned to eat healthier. or developed an exercise program)*

4. *What could you do now to improve on one of the condition(s)? (i.e., may be similar to answers in #3)*

7. **I like playing the role of the martyr.** I have heard a parent say to her children, "This is why I am sick. Look how you are behaving." or "I just do and do for others - it's too overwhelming" What this really translates to is "See, all I do for others. It is causing my illness."

The "martyr syndrome" is a term I coined to describe those who use their responsibilities or obligations to others as excuses for not improving their life and regaining their health. In Webster's dictionary a martyr is one "who makes a great show of suffering in order to arouse sympathy."

If we are serving and giving to others because we love them and we enjoy it, then our health will improve. But, on the other hand, if we are doing those things grudgingly, resentfully, or for sympathy from others for "**all** that we **have** to do" then we are playing the martyr. This kind of thinking and behavior can bring on a multitude of health conditions. We must either step out of ourselves in loving service to others, or we must let go of or delegate some of the responsibilities that are causing us to feel this way.

1. *What are the reasons you are doing so much for others? (i.e., guilt, attention, sympathy, love)*

2. *What are the feelings you experience while giving so much of yourself?(i.e., resentment, stress, tired, neglected)*

3. *Are you using the illness to reinforce to yourself and others that you're doing too much?(i.e. feeling that the illness is due to not getting enough rest because of others demands, or not having the time to take care of yourself)*

4. *What can you do now to relieve some of the burdens and stress you feel from caring for others and performing your obligations? (i.e .share responsibilities with another family member, make time for self, set limits on those things you can or can't do)*

5. *How are the people in your life perceiving or affected by your illness, time and effort spent in their behalf? (i.e. worried, effort is spent grudgingly, stressed)*

6. *How can you change your perceptions regarding the way you feel about dealing with your responsibilities? [i.e. family (serving out of love), job (choice to be here), commit-*

ments (choose a positive attitude)].

7. *What is the benefit you are receiving from the illness, and do you really want that kind of response or feelings from others? (i.e. sympathy from others, pity, guilt trip placed on others.)*

8. I don't have to give up my lifestyle. My great-grandfather died in the hospital from emphysema and lung cancer. Sadly, while underneath an oxygen tent, his last request was to have another cigarette. He had been willing to sacrifice his health for a lifestyle of an addiction that he brought upon himself. He had given power and control over to that negative vice that ended his life in a painful, suffering way.

Some people have the attitude, "Eat, drink, and be merry, for tomorrow we die". They have not been to a hospital, emergency room, or elderly care center where those who have lived an irresponsible lifestyle do not just "die tomorrow." Most of these people spend their last number of years dying, with pain, misery, discomfort, and the burden of knowing so many people had to care for them.

We don't know how strong or weak our constitution is until it is put to the test. Then it may be too late. While others may drink, smoke, eat a high-fat, high-sugar diet and seem to get away with it, that same lifestyle may affect us completely differently. I have heard others say, "Everyone has to die from something so why bother?" or "I'm just too busy to take care of myself." The bottom line is, "You can take the time now to be healthy or you'll **have** to take the time later to be sick." Eventually it will catch up to you.

Our lifestyles are affected by our social and family cultures, dietary habits, addictions, and work environments. When we choose not to give up those things that can negatively affect ourselves, (physically, mentally, emotionally, and spiritually) and our loved ones, we are basically saying, "I'd rather sacrifice my health than to sacrifice my lifestyle". The choice is always ours. No matter, we, and our loved ones, will have to live with it.

1. *Is your lifestyle really worth sacrificing your physical, mental, emotional, or spiritual quality of life?*

2. *How do you feel about the sorrow and burden that may end up being placed upon family or others by the unhealthy lifestyle choice(s)?(i.e. knowing they now must take on more responsibility or the sadness and hurt from a loss)*

3. *How can you manage your time in order to spend the necessary time on improving your own health? (i.e. prioritize the important commitments in life, change to a less demanding job, or change surroundings or people associated with)*

4. *What are some things you may have to sacrifice when making a healthier lifestyle change? (i.e. a social environment, popularity, friends, or job)*

5. *Would you like to have more power and control over own life? If yes, list the areas.*

6. *What are some things you enjoy doing that you could replace the negative or self-defeating behaviors with?(i.e. exercising, a new hobby, obtain more education)*

9. **I can just accept my fate.** A man in his late fifties with numerous health problems said, "My doctor says that this is how I'll **always** be so I just have to accept it." He felt that there was no point in trying to do things to improve his

health because they wouldn't work anyway. In other words believing that he had no choice, or that it wasn't his fault makes it is easier to just accept his fate. He then felt justified that he did not need to make any effort.

It's often easier to accept what someone tells us our life is going to be like than to try to take charge of our situation and see if there is any thing we can do to improve it. Especially when the opinion is given to us by someone we feel is competent, educated and has our best interest in mind. No matter what our condition, a positive attitude can encourage a healing process. Just as our thoughts and emotions can make us sick, they can also make us well. Miracles can happen when we do not allow someone else to designate our fate, but become the "captain of our own ship."

1. *List any condition(s) you have been told that you will just have to live with or accept. (i.e. overweight, depression, diabetes)*

2. *How could you educate yourself on the condition? (i.e. talk to others with the same condition, research alternative therapies from books, internet, or a competent health care practitioners)*

3. *What could you do, after researching the condition, to improve or eliminate the problem? (i.e. change dietary habits, move to a different location, change jobs, use an alternative therapy)*

4. *What are some ways to change your belief, attitude or perception about the condition? (i.e. become more educated on the condition, learn how to gain a more positive attitude, understand that there is always hope)*

10. **I can escape from my reality.** A married woman in her late thirties still rearing children, felt that the only way she could cope was to numb life experiences with drugs. She stated, "I don't want to be in reality because this (the effect of the substance) is a much more pleasant world to be in".

Often, we find people who are hurting (emotionally, physically, mentally, and spiritually) and are using not only their health problems, but drugs or alcohol to cope. The drugs become the crutch and the condition is the excuse. This then becomes a viscous cycle. We take the drugs to mask the problem, then we feel better for a while, then we start to feel bad, guilty or feel the hurt, then we take more drugs, etc. We can never heal ourselves if we are dependent upon chemicals.

The chemicals in our body are very sensitive and complicated. When we alter our body functions we have set ourselves up for serious chemical imbalances. These imbalances can affect our brain, emotions, physical health, and relationships. We haven't faced and dealt with the initial problem - we have only compounded it.

The first thing to do is to identify the reason for the "hurt". Is it physical, mental, emotional, spiritual? Whatever the cause, the drugs may help short term, but the side effects can be long term. The media is a big advocate of using drugs to solve our problems. Commercial after commercial tells us that we need drugs to function in life (i.e. "Come back to Prozac" or new drug uses for P.M.S). *(See Chapter 5 on Chemicals "Avoid exposure to toxic substances")*. There are many other healthier options to choose from if we just make the effort to try them.

1. What is the reality that is making you so miserable? (i.e., poor relationship with spouse, stress from children, discontentment with job, unhappy lifestyle, physical problem)

2. *What kind of control do you have over the unhappy or stressful situation? (i.e., could change jobs, seek marriage, or family counseling, learn new ideas for healthier lifestyles)*

3. *What options do you have to help eliminate this health condition? (i.e., find an alternative to drug therapy, improve diet, spend more time outside or exercising, seek a competent alternative health care practitioner)*

4. *Are the choices I'm making the most productive and beneficial way to cope my health condition?(i.e., using drugs to cope, not managing stress or anger appropriately, isolation from others)*

5. *Are any of my loved ones affected by my choice to escape from reality? If so, how are they affected?(i.e. frustration, resentment, irritability, lonely, angry, demands on time, overburdened)*

6. *Do I need help in eliminating the drugs/alcohol from my life? (i.e., addicted, dependent)*

7. *If so, where can I get the help? (i.e., community professional, church leaders, friends, family, support groups)*

8. *What will my life be like if I am drug/alcohol free and have dealt appropriately with my health condition? (i.e., peaceful, healthier, in control, able to solve problems and be a team player)*

SUMMARY OF THE BENEFITS AND NEW PERCEPTIONS

Finally, summarize the results of your responses from the various benefits with the following questions:

1. Are any of these benefits keeping you from making the effort to improve your health? If yes, then list the benefits and refer back to each individual benefit and review each response focusing on the positive ways to deal with the health concern.

2. How important is it to you to be independent, healthy, and in control of your life? What would you be willing to do or give up?

3. Are you willing to make the time and effort required to improve the quality of you and your family's life? If yes, how will you go about it?

4. Are your choices, behaviors, attitudes, or health conditions affecting yourself, your family or other important people in your life? If so, list the people affected and in what ways is each person affected?

5. Write down your goals and the steps you would need to take to improve your health and your home, work, church, or community environment.

THE HEALING PROCESS

People often ask us, "Can I just do some of the suggestions in this book? It is too hard to do them all." and our response is *"It depends upon how much health you want"*. The truth of the matter is that any positive change you make will improve your health and it will benefit you physically, emotionally, mentally, and spiritually. It is up to you how much improvement you want compared to how much time and energy you are willing to commit to.

So, do not feel overwhelmed or that you must do everything exactly right all at once or even all of the time. For some people it is easy to just decide today to make the necessary changes, whereas others need to take it one step at a time. Either way you will notice improved health and well being and you will feel more in control of your life. As our weaknesses become our strengths, we will then be in a position to help others in bringing health and happiness into their lives.

For many of you who strive to be healthy, wish to help someone else, there may be some tips for you through out this manual that will give you or a loved one more tools to continue on a healthy path. Wherever we are in life, we can always improve and progress one step further.

CHAPTER 2

IDENTIFY AND OVERCOME "STRESSORS" PREVENTING ULTIMATE HEALTH

ARE YOU FEELING "STRESSED OUT"?

It's 8:30 a.m. The bell rings and 30 young, energetic children come rushing through the door of a classroom to find their seats. Eagerly looking up from their desks, the students are waiting for their teacher's next move. The teacher quiets the students, takes roll, explains the rest of the day, and quickly gets started with the day's activities. The students begin working on with all of their energy and enthusiasm. The noise level in the room begins to escalate. Children's hands are rising in the air one by one bidding the teacher's attention.

Picture yourself as the teacher. How would you describe this experience – fun or stressful? We all have similar experiences. It's our perceptions of the experiences and our reactions to them that make the difference. What one person considers fun or a challenge, another considers stress. Stress can affect us more than we realize. It can make us miserable, anxious, depressed, worried, or even sick.

There are factors that can cause stress and can trigger many different complaints or illnesses. During our life, "stressors" (anything that can trigger a stress related response) can change. What may cause stress at one stage in life may not be cause of stress at another. For example, what may have caused you stress as a child (i.e. is anyone going to laugh at my new haircut?) may be different than what is causing you stress now (i.e. starting a new job), or in 20 years (i.e. being alone).

We can have power over the stressors in our life. We can learn to control our responses to them. We can learn to manage stress appropriately, as we understand some of the factors that can cause stress and how it can affect us. As you consider the following causes of stress, see if you can identify what areas are the most concerning in your life.

1. *Think back over the different stages of your and list the various stressors you can remember. Are they still causing you stress now?*

2. *Consider the future stages of your life and speculate as to what kind of stressors you foresee.*

FACTORS THAT CAN CAUSE STRESS

1. Lack of balance in our lives. Some of our stressors we have no control over (i.e. a bad choice made by a family member). We need to let go of the stressors we have no control over. Worrying will not change anything. We need to identify what is causing our life to be out of balance and then focus our energies on those stressors we do have control over.

1. *Try to identify an area(s) of your life that you feel may be out of balance and causing you stress (i.e., too much demand on time, job, family, trying to accomplish too much at once, or an unhappy a relationship)*

2. *What area(s) of your life do you have control over? What are some ways you can change them?*

2. Physical factors. Some may include the **misuse of drugs (legal or illegal), exposure to toxic substances (tobacco, alcohol, chemicals, additives, etc.), a poor diet, or a lack of**

exercise, water, or sleep. Maybe you can identify with any of these stress factors.

1. *List some of ways you could eliminate these stressors in your life. (i.e., change to a healthier diet, start an exercise program, obtain professional help for an addiction)*

2. *List the steps you would need to take to eliminate the stressors, and devise a plan to assist you as you approach this task. (i.e., research some of the foods that help to relieve the symptoms of stress, make an appointment with a competent health care practitioner, or sign up at a weight gym)*

3. **Family factors.** Family issues could be contributing to the stress in your life. Such factors could be: **fighting with another family member, moving to a new location, financial problems, abuse, a family member leaving home, behavior problems with children, health problems with a family member, a divorce, or death.**

1. *Write down how you feel any of these factors may be affecting you and / or your family.*

2. *Are any of these factors beyond your control? If so, we must be able to let go of the burden, frustration or anger we may feel and deal only with those stressors that we do have control over.*

3. *Are any of these factors within your control? If so, what could be some positive ways that you could deal with them? (i.e., holding a family council to discuss and resolve a problem, seek marriage counseling, or join a support during grieving)*

After writing the possible solutions down, prioritize beginning with the most important ones and begin working on them one at a time. By taking things one at a time, you will avoid unnecessary stress of trying to deal with too many problems all at once.

4. **Environmental factors.** Most environmental factors are beyond our control such as **natural disasters (floods, tornadoes, hurricanes, etc.), wars, noise, air, and water pollution.** Other factors include **extremes of temperature or humidity, lack of sunlight or excess sunlight, and traumatic accidents.** These factors can be devastating and recovery may take a long time. If any of these types of stressors play a role in your stress level, respond to the following questions.

1.   *Write down some ways that would help you and your family recover more easily. (i.e., moving to a new location, enlist the help of family or community members, brainstorm ideas to improve the situation)*

2.   *If moving is not an option, are there ways you could make your environment less stressful? If so, list them. (i.e., use an air or water purifier in your home, or adjust the times spent outdoors, check with community and health agencies for assistance)*

5. **Job factors.** Stressors can surface at work. They can include: **starting a new job, retirement, possibility of loss, too much work, poor relationship with the boss or other employees, unclear duties or responsibilities, or the job does not feel rewarding or satisfying to you.** Sometimes we feel trapped in a job and feel that there is no way out. These stressors can be reduced even if we are not in a position to change jobs right away.

1. *List the stressor(s) that you might be feeling.*

2. *List some ways you may be able to change your job situation. (i.e., gain more education, apply for a different position – either in the same company or a different one, make sure you have a written copy of the job description and discuss it in detail with your supervisor, improve your own communication skills, or look for ways to lessen your work load or become more efficient in what you are presently doing.)*

3. *Check with your local community or state college regarding their career center and the services they provide to the community.*

4. *Work with a career counselor. He/she may be able to show you new opportunities.*

5. *Take an interest, aptitude, and ability inventory. It may help you focus in an area that will be more rewarding and enjoyable to you.*

5. **Change.** We go along in our life feeling pretty comfortable. Suddenly, something happens to take us out of our "comfort zone." It could be our own choice or something we had no control over. Nonetheless, we experience stress. Change can occur in various areas such as: a **personal loss, an illness or injury, a change in lifestyle, a change in the family, a change in a relationship, or relocating to a new home.** Many of the situations previously discussed resulted in some form of change. Remember the saying, "The only thing that is constant is change." Change is inevitable. Learning to experience it and deal with it will greatly reduce our stress levels.

1. *Write down some of the changes that occurred in your*

life in the past year.

2. *Write down how you handled these changes and any suggestions to yourself on how you may have been able to handle them better.*

6. **Other stress factors.** **Biological stressors** include a host of diseases. **Social** stressors involve **relationships or lack of, activities either alone or with someone else.** Other stressors include **crime, racism, or wars.**

1. *List any of these stressors occurring in your life.*

2. *List ways you may be able to improve upon or handle them better. (i.e., find ways to improve your health, adopt a hobby, make sure your home or work is as safe and secure as possible)*

7. **Eustress.** This can be a positive form of stress in our lives usually keeping us on our toes. It helps us to stay motivated and do our best. Activities in our life that involve eustress stress include: **competitions, getting married, having a baby, going to college, and getting a promotion.** Without any form of stress in our lives we would be like a slug- not accomplishing much or moving forward with any desire to improve our lives. We need to be careful, though, that we do not fill our lives up with too much of this kind of stress or we end up with what is commonly called **burn out.** It can also be a negative stress factor depending upon our perception and reaction to the situation. Finding the right balance in our lives is critical.

1. *Identify any areas where you may be placing undue stress on yourself. (i.e. meeting deadlines, setting too many or too high goals, or making too many changes all at once)*

2. *List some ways to relieve or space out some of the events that are causing stress. (i.e. attend college part time instead of full time, or find ways to manage time more efficiently)*

REACTIONS TO STRESS

Top selling drugs in the United States are those used for depression and nervous disorders. This suggests that some of our major health problems relate to stress and emotional, physical, and behavioral factors that can cause it. In the 1991, *Stress Research* journal, an article estimated that about 60 percent of the visits to family doctors are brought forth by symptoms related to stress and emotions.

The stress of returning to a job you dislike on Monday morning can have a fatal outcome for a person at risk for a heart attack. "Black Monday Syndrome" is term coined for heart attacks that occur on Monday mornings between 7 and 9 a.m. More heart attacks occur on Monday than on any other day of the week. Job stress can affect us both physically and emotionally.

Our bodies respond to stress differently. The better you know yourself, the better you will be able to reduce the stress in your life. The following diagram depicts our response to stress in three major areas.

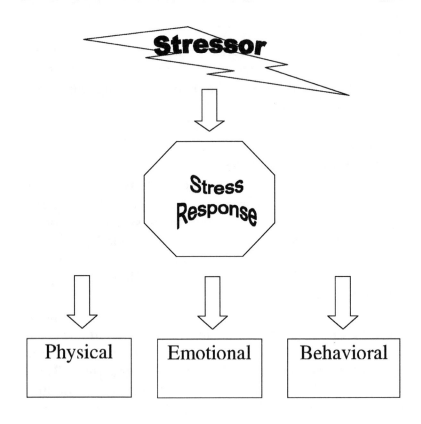

1. **Physical symptoms.** If stressors are not reduced or managed in a positive way, they can compromise our immune system and set up an environment for disease. Our immune system fights to protect our body against disease by seeking out and destroying harmful bacteria and viruses. When we are under stress, our body releases hormones (like cortisol and adrenaline) which can alter the way our immune system functions. Some **physical symptoms** of stress are:

headaches, stomach aches, back/neck/jaw pain, dizziness, ulcer sores on mouth or tongue, fatigue, inability to sleep or excessive sleep, weight loss or gain, high blood pressure, nervousness, change in appetite, hives, diarrhea/constipation, skin problems, crying, feeling ill, digestive disturbances, or heart palpitations.

If you can identify any of these symptoms at the onset, you may be able to prevent or lessen their effect. You may notice other symptoms of stress not mentioned. Everyone's body responds differently. These physical symptoms, if not dealt with appropriately, can turn into more serious health problems such as: heart disease, cancer, digestive problems, infectious diseases, respiratory illnesses, yeast and fungal infections, EBV, and arthritis.

1. *Write down any physical symptoms that your body experiences when you are under stress.*

2. *List any unhealthy ways you have dealt with these symptoms and the results.*

3. *Now list any healthy approaches you can or have used to address the problem. (i.e., taking a long walk, deep breathing, getting plenty of sleep, relaxation techniques, eating healthier, or taking a nap).*

2. Emotional symptoms. Some people suffering from stress can become fatigued, even to the point of malfunctioning. **Emotional symptoms** of stress include:

anxiety, hostility, irritability, loss of self-esteem, feelings of helplessness, withdrawal from others, loss of concentration, substance abuse, feeling pressured, moodiness, defensiveness, nightmares, panic attacks, thoughts of suicide, depression, restlessness, confusion, and aggressiveness.

We must accept the things we cannot change and let go of those we can't. How do you know if you have really let go? You don't say, "Yeah, but..." For example, "Yeah, but, he really hurt my feelings - last year!" The "Yeah, buts..." are those who no matter how rationally you try to explain to them about how they do not have any control over a situa-

tion and to accept it and then let it go, say, "Yeah, but..."!
They are still emotionally reacting to that particular stres-
sor.

We must learn to modify our responses to what we consider stressful situations. This does not mean to avoid activity or challenging situations. We must understand what types
of situations provoke us and avoid unnecessary irritations.
Write down any emotional symptoms you can identify with.

1. *List any stressors that may be causing emotional symp-
    toms.*

2. *Ask yourself the following questions, "Will this even
    matter next year?" "Is this really worth getting upset
    over?" or "Is this a truly threatening situation or just a
    annoying one?" By understanding the seriousness, or
    not, of the situation, we may be able to realize that it is
    not as important as we thought.*

3. **Behavioral symptoms.** These can be detrimental to our
overall health. When we are not dealing with stress in a positive way, we often turn to other avenues to help us cope.
Some of the avenues we choose may be annoying and frus-
trating - not only for us but others as well. There are **behavioral symptoms** of stress such as:

   **smoking, tardiness, nail biting, grinding teeth, clumsiness,
tapping, use of alcohol, drugs, or tobacco, compulsive dieting or compulsive overeating.**

   Avenues, like substance abuse, can harm us physically,
mentally, emotionally, and spiritually. The use of tobacco,
drugs (legal or illegal), and alcohol does not solve our problems - they only compound them and add more stress to our
lives. How stressful is it to try and break an addiction? How
stressful is it to deal with physical health problems brought
on by the use of any of these substances?

1. *List any of the behavioral symptoms you can identify with.*

2. *Write down how you feel they are affecting you and other important people in your life.*

3. *Prioritize the behavioral symptoms you want to change and make a plan to approach each one. (i.e., seek professional if needed, learn relaxation techniques, eat a healthy diet, or get plenty of rest)*

POSITIVE WAYS TO REDUCE OR ELIMINATE STRESS

Now that we have identified various stressors in our lives and how these stressors can negatively affect us, let's take a look at some positive ways to reduce stress. Remember, because of our perception of the activity, what works for one person may not work for another. You must find what works for you.

Nutrition plays a vital role in stress. When we are under stress our body becomes more acidic. An environment that is too acidic is more prone to disease. To help your body balance the acidic condition and relieve the stress related symptoms, there are certain things that you can do:

1. **Eat more alkaline forming foods** such as: fresh fruits, vegetables, sprouts, cereal grasses, garlic, and foods high in fiber. Soak whole grains and legumes before cooking them. Soaking starts the sprouting process which is alkalizing. Chew your food well to mix it with saliva which is an alkaline fluid. Eat plenty of Omeg-3 foods such as: flax seed and flax seed oil, soy foods, pumpkin seeds,

dark leafy greens, fish or fish oil, spirulina, seaweed, nuts and seeds.

2. **Avoid processed foods,** artificial sweeteners, carbonated drinks, junk food, fried food, red meat, sugar, white flour products, caffeine, alcohol and tobacco. Food and dairy allergies, and metal toxicity can show symptoms of stress.

3. **Adding supplements** to your diet may be beneficial. Try the B vitamins, Vitamin C and E, zinc, magnesium, and calcium. Some people have found CoQ10, L tyrosine, and melatonin to be helpful.

4. **Aromatherapy** using essential oils may be helpful for some people. Oils such as lavender, bergamot, chamomile, clary sage, geranium, and cypress are helpful in reducing the symptoms of stress. Essential oils can be diffused in the air, rubbed on the bottom of your feet, added to bath or shower gels, shampoo, massage oil, lotions or creams.

5. **Homepathic remedies** have been found to bring great relief to many. To be effective, the right remedy must be chosen based on symptoms and circumstances. You will need to do some research to find the right remedy for you. Some options are:

nux vomica – stress from over indulgence

kali phosphoricum-depression, anxiety, burned out from business or work

cocculus – stress over loved ones or others, loss of sleep, anger or grief

phosphoricum acidum – stess from grief or physical illness

calcarea phosphorica – deep depression, loss, boredom

magnesia phosphorica – cloudy thinking, irritable, over sensitive

adrenalinum – type A personality, pushes on no matter what

6. Herbs are great for relieving the symptoms of stress. Here too, you will need to do some research to find the one that may benefit you the most. Some herbs include: ginko biloba (brain function and circulation), milk thistle (liver cleanse), catnip (relaxant), chamomile (nerve tonic, digestion), Dong quai (supports the adrenals and nervous system), hops (nerves), kava kava (relaxant), ginseng (nerves, mental focus), valerian (nervous system), and St. John's Wart (antidepressant).

1. *List some of the nutritional items that you should consume more of and list the items you should avoid.*

2. *Make a plan outlining the new nutritional habits that you feel could benefit you.*

   *Herbs, supplements, and homeopathic remedies are to be used medicinally and on a short term basis until the symptoms subside.

The following is a list of ideas you may be able to apply to your situation and use in your life. You may be able to think of others not listed. If so, write them down. Design your own list that you can keep handy during stressful times.

TURNING STRESSORS INTO STRENGTHS

1. *Examine your attitude toward what is causing the stress. See if you can identify any positive aspects to the situation.*

2. *Learn to accept what you cannot change (until changing is possible).*

3. *Strike a good balance between work and recreation.*

4. *Involve yourself in an aesthetic experience – writing, painting, gardening, sculpting, music, etc.*

5. *Try meditating for a few minutes each day or using relaxation or visualization techniques.*

6. *Learn to say "No" to requests you cannot respond to.*

7. *Do not pin negative labels on yourself. ("I am...fat, scatterbrained, etc., as this becomes destructive self talk. It changes the mental programming in your brain. The "I am's..." can become a reality)*

8. *Be tolerant and forgiving of others - remember we live in an imperfect world.*

9. *Prioritize your responsibilities and commitments.- take one thing at a time.*

10. *Talk less, and listen more.*

11. *Get enough sleep and rest – lack of sleep causes you to become more irritable.*

12. *Eat healthy - stay away from refined foods, additives, and overly processed and high fat foods. Eat whole grains, fresh fruits and vegetables. Drink lots of water.*

13. *Avoid caffeine, alcohol, drugs, tobacco, and over eating.*

14. *Exercise 5 times a week for at least 20 minutes. It helps to relax muscles and reduces mental stress. This is also a way to find time for yourself.*

15. *Talk out your problems with someone you trust and who will not judge you.*

16. *Avoid self-pity. When you focus too much on yourself you can become more distressed. Try thinking of and doing more for others.*

17. *Learn from your experiences – so you won't repeat your mistakes.*

18. *Develop a positive disposition – it helps you to look at the bright side of things. What is the conversation that goes on in your head? Using a sense of humor helps you avoid the negative thoughts or taking things too seriously.*

19. *Give in once in a while. If you find the source of your stress is others, give in instead of fighting and insisting you are right.*

20. *Breathe deeply and often. When we are under stress, our breathing is very shallow.*

21. *Find a hobby that is different from your work. Do something each day you think is fun or that you love to do.*

Spend time outdoors.

22. *Stay away from others who are negative and who may bring you down.*

23. *Avoid procrastination. When we put things off, we think about them and they become stressful.*

24. *Become less competitive with yourself and others.*

25. *Ask yourself, "How much will this matter in a year?"*

26. *Think of solutions – not problems*

27. *Spend time with friends and family.*

28. *Learn to be organized by making a list or keeping a planner or appointment book.*

29. *Drive slower. Leave a few minutes earlier so you don't feel rushed. When you drive a little slower you are not as tensed about your own driving or others.*

30. *Believe that people have good intentions and are doing the best job they can.*

The following is a "Life Event Stress Test". If you decide to take it, keep in mind events in our life change from year to year - or day to day for that matter. If you find you score high, don't panic. You have learned some ways to help you relieve some of the stress in your life at this point. If you retake this test in six months or a year, your numbers will be different. Life is a series of changes –expect it!

LIFE EVENTS STRESS TEST

The following scale gives an estimate of the impact of the various stressors in a person's life. Consider these experiences that you may have had during the past 12 months. Add up the total of each of the experiences. If you scored below 150, you are about average in amount of stress you experience. You have a low chance of becoming ill. If you scored between 150 and 300, you have a greater chance of showing symptom of stress including illness. If you scored higher than 300, you have a higher risk of illness and changes in your health and /or behavior.

STRESS POINTS	SCORE
Death of a spouse	100
Divorce	73
Separation	65
Detention in jail, etc.	63
Death of a close family member	63
Personal illness or injury	53
Marriage	50
Fired from a job	47
Marital reconciliation	45
Retirement	45
Change in health/behavior of family member	44
Spouse or self becomes pregnant	40
Sexual difficulties	39
Gaining a new family member	39
Business readjustment	39
Change in financial condition	38
Death or major illness of a close friend	37
Change in different type of work	36
Change in number of arguments with spouse	35
Taking on a significant mortgage or loan	31

Foreclosure on a mortgage or loan	30
Changes in responsibilities at work	29
Child leaves home	29
Trouble with in-laws	29
Outstanding personal achievement	28
Move to another area	26
Partner begins or ceases work outside the home	26
Change in living conditions	25
Begin or cease formal education	25
Changes in personal habits (dress, manner, etc)	24
Trouble with the boss	24
Major purchases	20
Changes in recreation	19
Vacations with or visiting the family	19
Changes with friends	18
Changes in sleeping habits	16
Changes in number of family get togethers	15
Changes in eating habits	15
Social events	12
Caught in a lie	11

*Remember, these are only rough estimates. And what you may consider stressful, others may not. If you find that one or more of these experiences is still having a strong impact on you, and it has been longer than a year, then repeat the test for the events in the preceding year. Compare your scores. The higher the scores mean that you have an increased risk for stress related symptoms. By knowing this, you can start to look for ways to reduce the amount of stress in your life and therefore, lower you risk of symptoms.

CHAPTER 3
CONSISTENTLY STAY HYDRATED

DRINK UP!—

"WHO KNEW IT COULD BE SO SIMPLE?"

Picture a hot, dry dessert where the ground is hard, parched and cracking. It has not had consistent rain fall for a long time. Suddenly, it down pours. What does the water do? Not having ample time for the ground to absorb the water, it quickly runs off forming flash floods. But, if that rain continues, slow and steady, the ground will start to soften and soak up the water. The ground is no longer hard, dry, and cracked. At that point, a miracle happens. Vegetation begins to flourish. It becomes beautiful and healthy. And so it is with our body. Properly hydrated, we can receive the same wonderful benefits as the new desert. No more dry, cracked, dying cells – inside or out. The key to hydration is slow, steady, and consistent.

Water is the basis for life. It accounts for 65% or more of the weight of a healthy adult. It is the main component of all body fluids such as blood, lymph, digestive juices, tears, urine, and perspiration. We can live for weeks without food, but we can only live for days without water.

Consume 1/2 your weight in ounces of water each day on those days you are fairly sedentary. We lose approximately a pint of liquid each day just exhaling. Up the water intake to 2/3 your weight in ounces of water each day on those days which you are more physically active, eat a diet high in salt, or live in a very hot climate.

Water intake should be in small amounts. Your body absorbs about 4-8 ounces at a time. It you guzzle a large amount at once, the rest will be eliminated quickly-like the flash flood. Space the water intake to about every 20-30 minutes. At first, by increasing your water consumption you will also increase the number of trips to the rest room. After a while though, usually a few weeks, your body will start to absorb and metabolize the water and you will be eliminating less.

Try not to drink water immediately before, with or just after meals because it can dilute the digestive juices and reduce food digestion and the assimilation of nutrients. Be sure not to go to the extreme! If you drink too much water, you could reduce your electrolyte (important minerals) count.

The more you exercise, the more you need to drink. For every hour of strenuous exercise, you should drink about 24 ounces of water to keep your body fluid level in balance, and to increase your endurance and speed. Drink before you feel thirsty. Thirst is an inadequate indicator of hydration because a dry mouth is one of the **last** signs of dehydration. If you are exercising in cooler weather where you do not notice perspiration, you may not *feel* you are losing much water, but you still are.

Water should be purified and free from chemicals such as chlorine and fluoride. You can use distilled water while cleansing the body such as during a fast, being sure to take a good vitamin and mineral supplement.

Consume water that is at room temperature. It is hard on the body to drink very cold liquids. It can be hard on the heart because the cold liquid travels down along side it. It can also pull energy from the body trying to warm it up.

People often use tea (caffeinated), coffee, alcohol, and soda as part of their liquid intake. These products contain ingredients that can cause dehydration and leach important minerals from the body. You would need to drink one glass of water for every glass of one of these beverages just to keep the body fluid balance. Then you would still need to drink the required amount of water for your weight each day.

WATER'S AMAZING ATTRIBUTES

1. *Carries wastes and toxins out of the body. When wastes build up and store in the body we can become very toxic. We can damage our kidneys, bladder, and other organs because when the body rations water, our brain takes priority causing our other organs to suffer. This can lead to many diseases and health related problems. Water is a great solvent that helps to carry toxins out of the body keeping illnesses away. This means less colds and flu.*

2. *Facilitates the intake of oxygen and the excretion of carbon dioxide. If our lungs are moistened, we can take in more oxygen and get rid of more carbon dioxide. Oxygen inhibits disease whereas carbon dioxide is toxic to our body.*

3. *Prevents water and sodium retention. Water and sodium retention comes from not consuming enough water not from drinking too much. We have a misconception in our society regarding water. It is that in order to not retain water you must stop drinking it and /or use a diuretic. At first, if your body is not used to the new amount of water it may hold a little, but as it figures out that it will be receiving liquid consistently, it will let go of what it does not need. Our body tries try to retain what it is not getting enough of. When we take diuretics to try to eliminate water we are only dehydrating ourselves.*

4. *Speeds up our metabolism. Too little water can cause a sluggish thyroid and a slower metabolism. Toxins lodge in various glands and organs – especially the thyroid and can cause it to not function properly. This can cause weight gain because we are burning less calories. Purified water can remove toxins from the thyroid (especially distilled water).*

5. *Reduces or eliminates chronic conditions. Illnesses and chronic pain can be a sign of dehydration, especially if the pain is not related to an injury or an infection. Some typical problems linked to dehydration are: rheumatoid arthritis, headaches, constipation, colitis, heartburn, angina, high cholesterol, high blood pressure, and leg pain, allergies, urinary tract infections, hemorrhoids, asthma, varicose veins, and kidney stones. Try consistently upping your water intake to the suggested amount for a period of time before starting medications and see what the results are.*

6. *Flushes out excessive hormones. Stress and depression have been related to insufficient intake of water. When we are under stress or depressed our body releases various hormones and they become stored in areas of our bodies such as the kidneys. It takes water and exercise to flush the excess out of our system.*

7. *Reduces or eliminates low back pain. If you have low back problems water is crucial. When you become dehydrated, the intervertrebal discs and their joints are the first to be affected, especially the 5th lumbar disc. Drinking water replenishes the water stored in the disc core. This is the cushion needed for support and tension produced by muscle action.*

8. *Maintains good muscle function and tone. Water allows our muscles to contract easily without tearing. Your muscles can easily go into spasm if not well hydrated.*

9. *Lubricate the joints and tissues reducing soreness, stiffness, and damage. This is vital for athletes or people with health conditions such as arthritis.*

10. *Keeps our energy level up. We can lose speed and endurance when low on water. This can cause us to feel fatigued.*

11. *Keeps us youthful and alert with greater mental focus and clarity. Our cells are like sponges – they can hydrate and dehydrate. Once our body starts to absorb and metabolize the water, it finally reaches our cells keeping them pliable and producing energy. It also carries nutrients to the cells keeping them healthy and from shrinking. When it reaches our brain cells we become more alert. When it reaches our skin cells it keeps our skin from aging. Free radicals can damage our cells. Water removes free radicals that can result from dehydration.*

12. *Keeps our electrical system functioning properly. Water carries the electrolytes (sodium, chloride, potassium, calcium, and magnesium) to help convey electrical currents in the body. This helps prevent various nerve signaling problems.*

13. *Transports nutrients throughout our body. When nutrients are carried more efficiently through the body, we receive better assimilation and digestion.*

14. *Helps regulate the body's temperature. Perspiration helps us to dissipate heat thereby cooling the body.*

1. *Estimate how much water you and family drink each day?*

2. *Estimate how often do you or your family members drink water on a regular basis?*

3. *Are you or your family members showing signs of dehydration? List any.*

4. *What beverages would you need to reduce or eliminate in order to drink the appropriate amount of water each day?*

5. *Take a calculator and figure out how much water to consume each day. If your lifestyle is fairly sedentary, multiply your weight by 50%, if your lifestyle is active, multiply your weight by 60%.. This is the number of ounces of water to consume each day.*

6. *Find a container large enough to accommodate the water. If you only need to fill it once or twice a day, you won't have to think about how much water you are consuming. Sometimes it is hard to remember how many glasses of water you have already consumed.*

   *To prevent bacteria or infections, be sure to wash your container often and refill it with fresh, purified water.

CHAPTER 4

AVOID OR REDUCE CONSUMPTION OF ANIMAL PRODUCTS

IS "BETSY" REALLY A BLESSING?

Years ago, many people in our Western society felt that if they at least had "Betsy" – their milk cow - and plenty of meat, they would make it just fine during tough times. No one was too concerned about how much grains or fruits and vegetables they consumed each day. This wasn't the case for all cultures. Cultures such as the Native American, Eastern, Polynesian, etc. based their diet on whole grains with fruits and vegetables. They ate little or no meat or dairy products. Our modern illnesses were unheard of to them. They lived healthier and longer lives. It wasn't until the influence of the Standard American Diet (S.A.D.) that these cultures began experiencing the same common health concerns as our Western culture.

Although science has been able to extend our life span, in many cases the quality of life isn't necessarily what we had hoped for. Since heavily domesticating animals over the past few hundred years, our society has seen a rise in health problems such as: **gall bladder problems, chronic fatigue syndrome, candida overgrowth, kidney disease and stones, high blood pressure, arthritis, heart disease, strokes, diabetes, obesity, and cancer (especially of the bowel, prostate, breast, and lymphoma – cancer of the lymph nodes).** These diseases have been linked to a high fat, high-protein, and a high sodium animal-based (meat, poultry, fish, and dairy) diet.

We notice that in our culture people tend to think that colds, flu, tonsillitis, ear infections, bronchitis, allergies, etc. are part of every day life and we just have to live with them. Not necessarily so. By greatly reducing or eliminating animal products and eating a healthy, well-balanced diet, based on whole grains, and fresh fruits and vegetables, we can significantly reduce the number of common or seasonal illnesses.

SO WHAT'S THE BIG DEAL?

1. Products such as hot dogs, hamburgers, ham, sausage and other processed meats contain sodium sulfites, nitrites, nitrates, hog blood, skin, cereal, lungs, artificial flavors, colorings, preservatives and detergents. Meats also contain growth hormones, steroids, and antibiotics. Purchasing organically grown and fed animal products free of preservatives, additives, and other harmful chemicals can help reduce this problem. Besides being very toxic to our body, these products also hinder mineral absorption.

Dairy products contain hormones, antibiotics, and an excess of Vitamin D. Cheeses contain casein (also used to process glue) bleaches, dyes, mold inhibitors, synthetic flavorings, colorings, and preservatives.

2. Bacteria such as Salmonella, Listeria, and E-Coli, are a common contaminate of meat and dairy products. Sometimes we find fruits or vegetables contaminated too, but if you wash them well, we can avoid it. Often, we think we have caught a cold or the flu when in reality we have been contaminated with Salmonella or E-Coli because the symptoms can mimic each other.

3. Animal products contain saturated fat and cholesterol. Saturated fat is the fat that becomes solid at room temperature. This is the fat that clogs our veins and arteries leading to high blood pressure, high cholesterol, and heart disease. Immediately after consuming a high fat meal, our white

blood count increases, red blood cells become sticky and clump together instead of flowing freely like they should. Our body produces cholesterol on its own from the essential fats found in whole grains, nuts, seeds and other oil rich foods, so we do not need to consume it.

4. Compared to plant proteins, animal proteins contain more concentrated and larger molecules that absorb into the blood undigested and plug up our lymphatic (immune) system. If our lymphatic system cannot function properly and flush out toxins, bacteria, viruses, etc. out of the body, we end up with an environment for disease.

5. Animal products can cause an acidic condition in the body. The body tries to bring the acid/alkaline level back into balance by leaching calcium from the bones. This puts our bodies into a negative calcium balance. The more animal products we consume, the more calcium is leached out and eliminated through the urine. This is one reason why our society has such a high rate of arthritis and osteoporosis.

6. There is no fiber in animal products. We need fiber for proper digestion. Intestinal problems such as **colon cancer, irritable bowel syndrome** have been caused by a low fiber diet as have other problems like **frequent illnesses, flatulence, constipation, diarrhea and cramps.**

7. Dairy products are mucous forming. They can cause **allergic reactions, respiratory and digestive problems, sinusitis, slow metabolism, and mucous build up through out our entire system.**

8. Dairy products, especially cheeses, can cause a hardship on our glands especially our **thyroid, ovaries, prostate, tonsils and adenoids.** They can encourage **fibrous growths, kidney and bladder problems, and allergies.**

Women's bodies are more sensitive to dairy products. When women have eliminated the dairy products from their diets, the fibrous tissue in the breast becomes clearer and less dense, and cysts and other fibrous growths have vanished.

Weight loss occurs because the thyroid can function properly again,

9. Children are also very sensitive to dairy products. Some problems that have been linked to dairy products are **tonsillitis, allergies, congestion, lung problems, sleep problems, irritability, bed wetting, bronchitis, colic, frequent colds and flu, ear infections, and juvenile-onset diabetes.** In infants, a loss of iron and hemoglobin occurs and triggers blood loss from the intestines. The blood can often be seen in the stool.

GETTING THE ESSENTIAL NUTRIENTS

A frequently asked question is "Where do you get your protein and calcium?" Animals such as elephants or bulls do not consume meat or dairy. They grown large and strong from the nutrients found in plants. We can get all of the essential nutrients we need on a plant-based diet.

The following are 5 essential nutrients needed by the body for optimum health. *(see Chapter 6: Develop healthier eating habits for a more complete description of the following nutrients)*

1. Protein - You can find all of the essential amino acids required for human protein metabolism from **green vegetables, grains, legumes (peas, beans and lentils), tofu, and soy and nut milks.** It is not necessary to always worry about properly combining proteins at each meal. If you eat a variety of foods your body, especially the liver, will be able metabolize the protein and send out the needed nutrients. **Approximately 56 grams of protein for males, and 44 grams of protein for females per day. (Most people on the S.A.D consume around 100 grams - mostly from animal products!)**

2. Carbohydrates - Our body's energy needs are met by

consuming carbohydrates. Complex carbohydrates are packed full of vitamins, minerals, and fiber. They are naturally low in fat – a gram of carbohydrates has 4 calories compared to 9 calories in a gram of fat. Healthy food sources high in simple and complex carbohydrates are **grains, legumes, nuts, seeds, fruits, and vegetables.**

3. Fats - Essential fatty acids that we need are found in the oils of the **grains, nuts, and seeds (olive oil, flax seed, sunflower, etc)**, Always use cold or expeller-pressed oils and avoid products containing hydrogenated oil.

4. Vitamins and Minerals - **All fruits and vegetables grains, legumes, nuts, and seeds** contain and abundance of essential vitamins and minerals. One question that is often asked is "What about Vitamin B12 and calcium? Many products are fortified with vitamin B12 such as **soy, grains, nut milks, cereals., miso, tempeh, nutritional yeast, and fermented foods** . Fresh fruits and vegetables, even though they are rinsed, often contain small amounts of B12.

There are many great sources of calcium that are easily absorbed and used by the body. **Foods such as nuts and nut butters, seeds, leafy green vegetables, broccoli, lentils, dried fruits, carob, sea vegetables, and fortified soy and nut milks are excellent sources of calcium. You can replace dairy products with soy cheese, soy, grain or nut milks, and tofu.** Of course you can use B12 and calcium supplements if you are concerned that you may not be getting enough.

5. Water - Fruits and vegetables are considered high water content foods. They are not only building, but cleansing. If we are drinking the appropriate amount of water, and consuming plenty of fresh fruits and vegetables, we will acquire enough fluid in our body to keep it functioning optimally. (*See Chapter 3: "Consistently stay hydrated" for more*

information on the many other amazing attributes of water.)

BENEFITS OF REDUCING OR ELIMINATING ANIMAL PRODUCTS

1. **More economical.** 20,000 pounds of potatoes compared to 165 pounds of beef can be grown on one acre of land that will feed many more people.

2. **Healthier body.** We can **lower cholesterol, triglycerides, blood sugar and uric acid levels, and blood pressure; improve digestive problems; and reduce risk to cancer, diabetes, osteoporosis, and heart disease** due to the low-fat, high fiber diet. Generally, when we add more plants to the diet, we deliver more nutrients, antioxidants, and phytochemicals to our body. This will give us more energy and stamina. You can reduce or eliminate medications associated with these health problems.

You can improve, reverse, or prevent chronic inflammatory diseases such as: **arthritis, asthma, and eczema. Allergies, skin, joint, bowel, and glandular problems, osteoporosis, and PMS have subsided.**

3. **Stronger bones.** The calcium consumed from plants does not encourage calcium loss, as does the calcium from animal products. We absorb and assimilate all of the calcium.

4. **Weight loss.** Generally, once you stop eating animal products (and exercise regularly) those "unwanted pounds" melt right off. Even though you may be consuming more calories per day, you will be leaner. 1000 calories of vegetables and whole grains will not produce the amount of fat in your body as will 1000 calories of animal products.

One thing to consider is that men generally seem to have an easier time losing weight than do women. This is primarily because women's bodies genetically require more body fat because of the metabolic processes involved in creating the female hormones such as estrogen. So for women, "Be patient. It will eventually let go of the extra fat once the body realizes it does not need as much."

See Chapter 8: "Maintain ideal weight" for weight loss tips and information.

5. Eat more food! This is great plus for those of us who love to eat. So many diets cause us to feel deprived, unsatisfied, even angry or depressed. When you see how much food you can eat containing the same amount of calories as a regular meal in S.A.D., you will be amazed. **Eating becomes fun and exciting – not a guilt trip!**

6 LEVELS OF A PLANT BASED DIET

We follow a vegetarian-mostly vegan way of eating. People often ask me if we eat fish or eggs. Sometimes it is confusing when people say they are a vegetarian and eat eggs while others do not. There are many types of diet modifications you can make when choosing to reduce or eliminate animal products. The following explanation of the 6 levels of a plant-based diet should help to simplify this confusion

1. *VEGETARIAN – eats a plant-based diet*

2. *OVO-LACTO VEGETARIAN – eats dairy and eggs, but no meat, fish, or poultry*

3. *LACTO-VEGETARIAN – eats dairy, but no eggs, meat, fish, or poultry*

4. *OVO-VEGETARIAN – eats eggs, but no dairy, meats, fish, or poultry*

5. *FRUITARIAN – eats only fruits, seeds, and nuts*

6. *VEGAN – strictest of all vegetarian diets; no animal products at all*

    If you decide not to choose any of the levels of a plant-based diet, you can still receive health benefits by reducing the amount of animal products you consume each day/week. Depending upon the level of commitment you are willing to make, and the amount of improved health you want, choose what is right for you and/or your family.

    Research has shown that the VEGAN lifestyle is the healthiest of all levels; providing that the diet is based on whole grains, fresh fruits and vegetables. The FRUITARTIAN lifestyle has the most concerns with getting enough of the essential nutrients.

    Dr. Michael J. Klaper his book <u>A Diet For All Seasons,</u> stated a quote that I feel sums up why it is so important for us to take great care in choosing the foods we eat. He said" *…you are what you eat" (as well as* "who *you eat" – and what* they *ate!) "*

1. *How many times a day do you consume animal products? Week? Month?*

2. *Would you consider reducing or eliminating animal products from your diet? If yes, how would you go about reducing or eliminating the animal products? (i.e. each week add one more vegetarian meal to replace one containing meat, subscribe to vegetarian cooking magazine, purchase cook books, try to modify favorite recipes, look for meat/dairy substitutes)*

3. *What substitutions would you enjoy eating as replacements for the meat and dairy products? (i.e beans and legumes, meat substitutes such as soy or veggie burgers, TVP, soy cheeses or soy and rice milks)*

See "A New Hope for Health" *cookbook series for recipes that are meat and / or dairy free.* These cookbooks contains substitutions for meat, dairy, and egg products you can use with the recipes in the books or with your own recipes. Other cookbooks are in process.

I Love to Eat – Vegetarian!
I Love to Eat-Mexican!

CHAPTER 5

AVOID EXPOSURE TO
TOXIC SUBSTANCES

THE GOOD, THE BAD, AND THE UGLY

A number of years ago, I was a member of a small singing group. One evening, after a singing engagement, we went to a local Chinese restaurant. One of the women asked the waiter if there was MSG (monosodium glutamate) in the food. He assured her that there wasn't. We finished our meal and headed over to our motel. It wasn't long after we arrived that this same woman had a severe asthma attack. From previous experiences with MSG, she was sure that that was what had triggered it. We called the manager of the restaurant and explained our situation. He said that they use MSG in their sauces, but that when people request not to have it, they just don't add any extra to their dish.

Daily we are exposed to toxins – any agent that produces a harmful reaction in a biologic organism. Toxicity can come from food additives and preservatives, environmental contamination (such as pesticides and herbicides, air and water pollution), drugs, and pathogens (bacteria, parasites, molds/fungus, viruses). Reactions can range from mildly annoying to life threatening depending on a person's sensitivity. We can experience conditions such as fatigue, headaches, digestive problems, chronic conditions such as arthritis, autoimmune, candidiasis, hypertension, and cancer.

FOOD ADDITIVES AND PRESERVATIVES

A friend of mine was having a very difficult time with hyperactivity in two of her children. Not only when they were at home, but also when they were in school. The doctor wanted to put both of her children on Ritalin. She decided to see if there was anything she could do at home first. One at a time, she tried eliminating then adding various foods to their diet. She noticed that when the children consumed foods that contained colorings, especially red, they were much more hyperactive. She even noticed how the red coloring put in children's antibiotics caused this same reaction. She began buying and cooking with whole foods instead of processed. It was an amazing discovery for her. Her children did not need to be medicated.

Not only are highly processed foods high in fat and calories, and low in nutrients and fiber, they are filled with many additives and preservatives. Additives are usually flavorings, colorings, or substances that help to enhance the nutritional values of food that have been lost during processing. Preservatives help to extend the shelf life and prevent contamination and spoilage.

Many additives and preservatives have not yet been thoroughly tested for safeness. As in the red food coloring example, no matter how small the amount, even those that may be considered somewhat safe may cause a toxic reaction in someone who may be sensitive or allergic to that particular substance.

Although some people may have a toxic reaction to natural additives and preservatives such as corn syrup, sugar, mustard, salt, or vitamins, we will be focusing on common synthetic substances.

ADDITIVES

1. **Antibiotics** - They are found in most animal products and are administered to the animals in their feed and drinking water. Antibiotics are used to prevent disease, to stimulate the growth of young animals, and to increase egg production.

Found in – beef, pork, poultry, fish and dairy products

Side effects – you can experience the side effects of an allergy to an antibiotic such as hives, arthritis, fever, rash and headaches. They can cause an overgrowth of fungus (i.e. candida), swelling, irregular heartbeat, lupus, and antibiotic-resistant bacteria. They break down the friendly bacteria (acidophilus) in the colon.

2. **Aspartame** – Also known as NutraSweet, Equal, and Spoonful, aspartame is the most common synthetic product used today. It is used as a sugar substitute. It is similar in composition to MSG. It is considered one of the most deadly toxins in our society because of its presence in thousands of foods.

Found in – diet products, antibiotic syrups, chewable vitamins, Jell-O, and Kool Aid

Side effects – some include: swelling, headaches, weight gain due to the increased appetite (especially carbohydrate cravings), destroys brain cells, depletes serotonin from the brain, seizures, depression, memory loss, gradual loss of vision and eye problems, heart palpitations, menstrual problems, slurred speech, fatigue, irritability, insomnia, loss of equilibrium, and vertigo. Aspartame can by passed directly on to the fetus. Some diseases have been triggered by aspartame such as: Multiple Sclerosis (MS), Fibromyalgia, and Chronic Fatigue symptoms due to the methanol toxicity, cancer, tumors, epilepsy, diabetes, lymphoma, Alzheimer's, Parkinson's, and death.

3. **Fat Substitutes** - People enjoy eating high fat foods but usually do not want the extra fat and calories. A newer product, Olestra, is considered to be the answer, but has already been shown to cause severe problems.

Found in - high fat processed foods such as chips

Side effects - digestive problems, diarrhea, cramps, inhibits the body's absorption of needed carotenoids such as betacarotene, and fat-soluble vitamins such as A, D, E and K. Becoming deficient in these important nutrients can lead to such chronic diseases as cancer and heart disease.

4. **Food Colorings** - FD&C are food coloring additives found in process foods. They are mostly synthetic dyes. For years they have been considered toxic and carcinogenic and many have been banned. The most common and the most concerning are Yellow No.5 and Red No.40.

Found in – highly processed foods, especially those geared to children.

Side effects – asthma attacks, hives, hyperactivity (AD/HD), tumors in animals

5. **Hormones** - Hormones are given to animals to make them grow bigger and faster and to dairy animals to increase milk production. They are administered to the animals under the skin of the animal's ear.

Found in - beef, pork, poultry, fish, dairy products

Side effects - raised hormone levels in humans that may lead to hormone-related problems in females, aggression (especially in men), and early puberty

6. **Hydrogenated Fats** -Hydrogenated fats are trans-fatty acids produced by the process of hydrogenation. Hydrogenation uses hydrogen to solidify oils at room temperature. Purchase cold or expeller pressed oils such as

olive, flax, sunflower, soybean, canola, almond, peanut, etc.
    Found in – crackers, chips, margarine, shortening and fried foods
    Side effects - digestive problems, gall bladder problems, increased LDL blood cholesterol, and heart disease

7. **Monosodium glutamate (MSG)** - Derived from the Japanese Kombu plant, and now in its synthetic form, MSG stimulates the taste buds so we think the food tastes better. It is probably the most common of the flavor enhancers. It comes in powder and liquid form. The liquid form being more toxic to the brain because it is absorbed faster and produces higher blood levels.
    Processed foods containing glutamates such as: hydrolyzed vegetable protein, disodium guanylate, etc., must be labeled. Hydrolyzed vegetable protein is nothing more than high glutamate waste vegetables from other food processing and boiled in sulfuric acid.
    Found in - processed foods, salad dressings (especially Ranch), chips, frozen dinners, diet drinks, soups, fast foods, ethnic foods, gourmet foods, and condiments. In additives listed on the label which read: hydrolyzed vegetable/plant protein, sodium caseinate, calcium caseinate, yeast extract, textured protein, autolyzed yeast, plant protein extract, kombu extract..
    Side effects – headaches, asthma attacks, dizziness, chest pain, diarrhea, mood changes, sleep problems, hyperactivity, nausea, sweating, destroys nerve cells and the endocrine system, creates brain lesions, is linked to degenerative diseases (Alzheimer's, Parkinson's, etc), it causes the hypothalamus to secrete too much reproductive hormone, and can cause cardiac distress.

    8. **Saccharin** – has been the most controversial additive. It has been proven to cause cancer in animals, and it still

requires warning labels for foods for human consumption. Found in – diet products as a sugar substitute. Side effects – cancer in animals and questionable still for humans has been the most controversial additive. It has been proven to cause cancer in animals, and it still requires warning labels for foods for human consumption. Found in – diet products as a sugar substitute. Side effects – cancer in animals and questionable still for humans

PRESERVATIVES

1. **BHA** (butylated hydroxyanisole) and **BHT** (butylated hydroxytouluene) - These are used to prevent fats in foods from oxidation and rancidity. They also block access of oxygen to nutrients, which destroys the life of the food.

Found in – fatty processed foods, such as chips, or crackers. Also, found on packaging as on cereal boxes causing children to be more exposed.

Side effects – cancer in animals, hives, skin rashes and can trigger seizures

2. **Nitrites and Nitrates** - The sodium salts of nitrate and nitrite are used to cure and preserve processed meats. They help to control botulism, which is common among some cured meats. They also keep meat from turning brown. When added to foods, they can become cancer- causing chemicals known as nitrosamines. High temperature frying, as in bacon, can cause the worst of the chemical reaction.

Found in – processed meats (bacon, bologna, hot dogs, etc), sometimes found in drinking water, fruits and vegetables (not as significant amounts) grown in areas where the groundwater is contaminated and where there has been used an excess of synthetic nitrogen fertilizers.

Side effects – certain types of cancer (especially stomach), heart problems, sweating, lethargy and mental confusion

3. **Sulfites** - They were used to keep fruits and vegetables in restaurants and on salad bars fresh. In 1986, The Food and Drug Association (FDA) banned them for this purpose. They are still in use today.

Found in – peeled potato products, food packages (sulfur dioxide), dried fruit, seafood products, and wine.

Side effects – destroys vitamin B, can cause severe reactions in asthmatics, and death.

1. *Estimate the daily percentage of processed foods you/your family eat that contain additives or preservatives?*

2. *List any noticeable side effects these products are causing you or your family? (digestive problems, headaches, AD/HD, etc.)*

3. *What are some ways you could reduce the amount of processed foods containing additives and preservatives? (i.e., cook more from scratch, buy fresh fruits and vegetables, read labels carefully)*

ENVIRONMENTAL CONTAMINATION

A middle-aged woman was complaining about pain under her arm and suffering from constant flu symptoms. Years ago she had been bitten under the arm by a poisonous spider. She, along with her physician, felt that her symptoms were still related to the toxicity of the spider. She tried everything suggested, but the symptoms would not subside. Finally, she sought the help of another physician. He told her that he knew exactly what her problem was. About 25 years ago, she had had breast implants put in. The physician said that she was experiencing toxicity from them. She decided to have them removed. Within a couple of weeks her pain and flu symptoms vanished. She couldn't believe the difference in how she felt.

Environmental contamination can come from the air we breathe; the water we drink; the products sprayed on our foods, used around our homes, on or in our bodies; and exposure to heavy metals. Realizing that we do not have much control over the air we breathe, we can use air purifiers in our home if we live in a polluted area. The same goes for water. A good water purifying system will eliminate chemicals such as chlorine and fluoride. We can purchase organically grown food; and natural cleaning supplies pesticides, hair, skin, and nail care products.

1. Water

Fluorine is a gas used in aluminum manufacturing and the nuclear industry. The by-product or waste from this processing is Sodium Flouride. Sodium Flouride is added to our drinking water, most toothpaste's, and is used as rat and cockroach poison. It has been shown to promote certain cancers, ADD / ADHD (due to its affect on the brain)

Chlorine is used in water treatment plants to kill microorganisms that cause diseases such as hepatitis, cholera and polio. It is also used in bleaching flour and along with other chemicals destroys carotene and vitamin E. Chlorine kills the friendly bacteria in the intestines. It can cause acne, an overgrowth of candida, and cancer (especially bladder).

2. Foods and Home Products

Organically grown foods are sometimes more expensive to buy because they are more labor intensive to grow and produce. Organically grown foods are more nutritious, healthy, and safe. The reduced number of medical visits is worth the increased cost of the food.

Although the F.D.A. may restrict the use or tolerance of

some chemicals, we still consume enough chemicals in our foods to cause toxic reactions such as allergies, asthma, headaches, and chronic diseases. Other countries have fewer restrictions on chemicals used on foods than does the United States. If we purchase food grown out of the country, we are at a higher risk for exposure to toxic chemicals.

If you grow your own food, and wish to fertilize or use pesticides, be sure to use organic fertilizers and safe pesticides. By composting, you will grow healthy plants that will be strong enough to fight off infestations and disease.

In our homes we can use non-toxic products such as natural cleaning supplies and insecticides. Choose non-aerosol cans over aerosol. Stay away from solid and aerosol air fresheners. They contain chemicals that are known to be carcinogenic. Avoid household disinfectants containing the phenol or cresol.

3. Beauty aides

Skin, nail, and hair care products, and cosmetic surgeries are among the common beauty aides and are a growing trend in our society. They can cause severe reactions and toxicity in our body. Read labels and be aware of the product's ingredients we use in and on our bodies.

Avoid products containing synthetic ingredients, sodium lauryl sulfate, barium, mineral oil, alcohol, zirconium, aluminum, titanium and any words containing the word "prop" as in propylene glycol, or isopropyl alcohol. Even tattoo ink can leach into the bloodstream for years and cause toxicity.

There are many common cosmetic alterations using various chemicals and surgical methods. Procedures such as chemical peels, dermabrasion, and laser surgery can be very toxic. Our skin is like a large sponge and can draw in substances we place on it. They can also cause infections, scarring, skin allergies, fever blisters, and permanent damage or lightening of the skin.

Liposuction is the most popular cosmetic procedure and it causes the highest incidence of complications and death. One serious side effect is the damage done to the lymphatic system. Not only is fat removed but also blood vessels and lymph. When the lymphatic system is compromised the result is swelling and toxicity because the lymphatic system cannot remove the toxins as efficiently. Other serious side effects may be: infection, blood or lymph clots, edema, perforation of organs, bleeding, rippled or baggy skin and death.

Artificial implants include chin, cheeks, jaw, calf, and pectoral with breast being the most common. The implants are made out of silicone elastomer (rubber) that contains small amounts of various smaller silicones, metals such as tin and platinum, trace amounts of industrial chemicals, and large amounts of powdered silica. Implants are filled with a silicone or saline solution.

A new illness categorized by physicians now treating women with implants is called Silicone implant disease (also called human adjuvant disease or silicone-induced illness). Silicone is difficult to detox (rid) out of the system. The first step is to remove the implants. Once the implants are removed, there are products available on the market that will then help to rid the body of the stored silicone.

Side effects of implants can include: infection, hardening of scar tissue around the implants, nerve damage, severe weight loss, hair loss, liver problems, lymph node swelling and pain, chronic fatigue, circulation problems, arthritis pain, autoimmune symptoms, chronic muscle pain and stiffness such as back, shoulder, and neck. The body can develop antibodies that will attack collagen.

4. Heavy metals
Exposure to heavy metals such as mercury and aluminum can come from drinking water, foods, dental ware and cooking utensils. Mercury (amalgam) dental fillings have

been around for many years. Aluminum can be found in deodorants, antacids, baking soda and cookware. Some people have had severe reactions such as: nervousness, loss of memory, loss of attention, anxiety, insomnia, oral cavity disorders (bleeding gums, foul breath, gingivitis, etc.), gastrointestinal problems, cardiovascular problems headaches, dizziness, fine tremors (hands, feet, lips, eyelids, etc.) muscle problems, and cancer. Aluminum has now been associated with Alzheimer's disease.

There are many products on the market that are environmentally safe. You can also make your own products if you wish. *Check out your local health food stores for ideas. Read* <u>*The Healthy Home*</u> *by Linda Mason Hunter for natural products.*

Let's now consider some ways we can improve our immediate environment and reduce our exposure to toxic substances.

1. *List some ways you could clean up your environment and reduce our exposure to toxic chemicals (ie. replace metal dental fillings with healthier materials, install a water purification system in your home).*

2. *Identify some healthy alternatives that would improve your appearance and self-image (i.e. exercise program, nutritional supplements, improving your diet.)*

DRUGS

A frustrated mother came into my office because her son was causing problems in school and refused to take his AD/HD prescribed medication. The son's complaint was that the drug was causing him to feel very angry and he would lose his temper and start kicking walls or other objects. The mother also noticed violent mood swings along with a nervous tic that he had acquired.

As I continued to meet with parents and students, I began to pay close attention to the number of students who had been diagnosed with Tourette's Syndrome. Each time I asked the parents if the student had ever been on any AD/HD type medication. Out of about 10 cases, all but one said that the child had been. I started researching this and discovered that among all of the other side effects of these drugs, there is a possible neurological side effect.

Drugs can affect the brain, emotions, nervous system, cardiovascular system, and glandular system. They are not only prescription and over –the-counter medications, but other substances as well.

1. **Caffeine** is considered a drug. Although there are no restrictions on its purchase or use, it can cause adverse reactions in the body. Children are more susceptible to all forms of drugs and chemicals and therefore, caffeine should be avoided. Caffeine inhibits an important enzyme Phospho-diesterage (PDE) that is involved in the process of learning and memory development. Therefore, it is even more important to avoid if you are learning disabled or have a condition such as Alzheimer's disease.

Caffeine has been linked to fibrocystic breast disease. It pulls calcium from the body and excretes it through the urine. It irritates the liver and can settle in various places in the body including the brain. People think that caffeine gives them a boost of energy but the opposite is true. The body uses up its energy trying to get the caffeine quickly out of the system. This feels like a rush of energy, but in reality it is the body wasting its own energy in dealing with it.

Caffeine can cause nervousness, increased heart rate, irregular heartbeat, dilation of the blood vessels, high blood pressure, insomnia, birth defects from damaged chromosomes, diabetes, blood sugar level imbalances by forcing the pancreas to secrete too much insulin, kidney disease, calcium loss, dehydration, depression, gastric ulcers by increasing stomach acid secretion, digestive problems, cancer of the pancreas, insomnia, ringing of the ears, and addiction. It can also destroy the acidophilus in the colon.

2. **Anti-Depressants** such as Prozac, Zoloft, Paxil, Luvox, Effexor, and Serzone, are the most common of these types of drugs prescribed today. They are very powerful mind-altering drugs. They raise the cortisol levels in our body that can damage our liver, kidneys, and muscles. They can retard linear growth in children, who are more sensitive to the side effects of drugs, yet children from the ages of 6-12 are using them. Some of the serious side effects possibly linked to these drugs are mania, aggression, autism, anxiety, depression, mood disorders, nightmares, migraines, irritability, and compulsions for other drugs and alcohol.

People who consume diet products containing aspartame can experience the symptoms of depression, insomnia, fatigue, and irritability. These symptoms lead doctors to diagnose mental disorders. These and other mind, mood, and personality altering drugs are prescribed for these symptoms. Between the aspartame and the drugs, the chemical imbalances in the body are magnified so the symptoms compound themselves.

3. **Stimulants** are medications such as Ritalin, Aderol, Concerto, and their related psychiatric drugs. They are mind/personality altering drugs and are generally given to children and some adults who are diagnosed with Attention Deficit / Hyperactivity Disorder (AD/HD). Their use has increased over 600% in the last decade. AD/HD is a display of biochemical imbalances that can be improved by cleaning

up the child's diet and environment. These types of drugs have been linked to the stunting of a child's growth, aggression, mood swings, depression, insomnia, liver damage, and neurological disorders such as facial tics, and Parkinson's Disease.

4. **Antibiotics** as discussed previously under "additives", not only are we getting them in our foods, but there is also an overuse of them for medical treatment. Some side effects include hives, arthritis, fever, rashes and headaches. Other side effects may be an overgrowth of fungus (i.e. candida), swelling, irregular heartbeat, lupus and antibiotic-resistant bacteria.

Autism is now being looked at due to overuse of antibiotics. Antibiotics destroy not only the bad bacteria, but also the good. When this happens, it leaves our immune system weakened and more susceptible to various diseases.

5. **Alcohol** is a central nervous system depressant, and can act as a tranquilizer and a mild anesthetic. It is also an emotional suppressant that can lead to chronic depression. It is a toxic irritant to the body. It contains the mold ergot (a grain fungus – usually rye). The alcohol and mold reacts together making each even more toxic.

Some common problems are: inhibits calcium absorption, worsens P.M.S. symptoms, obesity, hepatitis, cirrhosis, allergy symptoms, pancreatitis and gallstones, gastric ulcers, hypoglycemia, diabetes, nerve and brain dysfunction, chronic infections (flu, cold, pneumonia, etc.), nutritional deficiencies (which can lead to a multitude of health problems), candidiasis, birth defects, impotence, coronary disease and many forms of cancer.

Even though some may argue that a small amount of alcohol, especially wine, helps to reduce the risk of heart disease, it can increase the risk of cancer. It is a flavonoid named

Quercitin found in grapes that help to prevent heart disease. So, if you want the extra the protection for your heart, drink grape juice or eat the grapes (especially red). Grapes will also help to prevent cancer. You will get double the benefit.

6. **Nicotine** intake is mostly through the use of tobacco – especially smoking. It is the single greatest cause of preventable disease. It is a nervous and cardiovascular system stimulant. Nicotine is not the only problem associated with cigarette smoking and tobacco chewing. Other problems are due to the thousands of carcinogenic chemicals concentrated in the tobacco.

The use of tobacco can lead to coronary disease; arteriosclerosis (by raising blood fat levels); strokes; lung diseases/cancer; chronic infections such as colds, flu, bronchitis, pneumonia, emphysema; asthma; many forms of cancer; allergies; nutrient deficiencies; Alzheimer's disease; varicose veins; senility; impotence; and rapid aging of the body – especially the skin.

Although tobacco is the most difficult addiction to break of the commonly used drugs, it is not impossible. People quit smoking everyday. A diet modification can help a person quit smoking. Eat whole grains, fresh fruits and vegetables, use cleansing herbs, and drink plenty of water. Avoid foods such as red meat, dairy, fried foods, sweets and refined products. Add more exercise to the daily routine to help clean out the body and replace the habit with a more constructive activity.

7. **Immunizations** or vaccines have reduced the epidemics of childhood infectious diseases, but now there is a great rise in the epidemics of chronic diseases. There has been a drastic increase in the occurrences of asthma, autoimmune diseases, mental disorders (including ADD/ADHD), mental retardation, and learning disabilities, seizures, autism, and an outbreak of the same condition that the vaccine is supposed

to prevent. The main vaccines to consider are the DPT, MMR, hepatitis B, polio, Hib, and chicken pox.

Besides these, there are many vaccines being produced and are being given to our small babies who have not had sufficient time to develop their immune systems.

This is a very controversial issue and it would be wise for a parent to investigate the necessity and the side effects of the various vaccines.

1.   *List the drugs you/your family are currently taking.*

2.   *List any noticeable side effects.*

3.   *Identify healthy alternatives for these drugs. (i.e herbal supplements, homeopathic remedies, or diet modifications)*

4.   *If a family member has an addiction to any of these drugs, how can you overcome it? (i.e. professional help, or support systems)*

5.   *Write down your goals and steps you must take remove toxic substances from you/your family's environment.*

PATHOGENS

Talk to a professional colon therapist about human worms or parasites and he/she will have some amazing stories to tell. One colon therapist I know had a client who constantly complained of intestinal problems, fatigue, and a general feeling of ill health. She decided to do a series of colonics. After about the 4th or 5th colonic a 2- foot tapeworm was expelled from her body. It was quite a shock for her to see something like that. She quickly began to feel better and took the necessary precautions to avoid this situation again.

Parasites, bacteria, viruses, and molds and fungus occur naturally in the body. When our immune system is functioning optimally, our body will keep a check and balance system to keep everything under control. The problem arises when, given the right environment, they become disease producing agents or "pathogens". Pathogens cannot survive in a healthy, clean, and toxin free body.

Often when we have pathogens living in our body or when we destroy them, their residual effects can also make us very toxic – either by what they have been eliminating or the decaying process after they die. If we have used drugs to destroy a pathogen, there are also side effects and residual effects from that drug. When we take antibiotics, we not only destroy the harmful bacteria but also the good bacteria that are part of a healthy immune system. The drugs weaken our immune system making it harder to fight off the next occurrence. It is best to use more natural methods, when possible, to build our immune system while destroying the harmful pathogen.

1. Parasites generally live in the digestive tract and survive by obtaining shelter and food from decaying matter off of another organism or "host"-us. The most common include the liver fluke, pinworm, tapeworm, roundworm (ascaris), and hookworm.

We can become infected from water, food-raw/uncooked, animals –usually those that live in the house, dirt, and other people with poor hygiene. They are everywhere. If we are healthy, have a clean body and intestinal tract, and have a strong immune system, parasites cannot live and when we are exposed to them they will pass quickly through our body without us even realizing they were there. When we are toxic, unhealthy, or have a weakened immune system, the environment is ideal for them to stay, build a home, and wreak havoc on our body.

Some symptoms of parasite infection include food cravings – especially to sweets, grinding teeth, nail biting, nose-picking, a large appetite, headaches, weakness, fatigue, digestive problems and even more chronic diseases such as Multiple Sclerosis, diverticulitis, chronic fatigue, or cancer. To help avoid parasite infection, here are some ideas: Eat raw brown rice, fresh garlic or onion, apple cider vinegar, pumpkin seeds, and drink a lot of water. To remove parasites from produce, soak fresh fruits and vegetables in a solution of ? cup apple cider vinegar or ? cup 3% food grade hydrogen peroxide in a sink full of water for 5-15 minutes. Rinse well. Cook animal products thoroughly.

2. Bacteria are small microorganisms such as listeria, e.coli, salmonella, staphylococcus, and streptococcus. Bacterial infections are often very painful. They can also make us sick with flu like symptoms such as diarrhea, vomiting, cramps, fever, and chills. Severe complications to bacteria infections can result in blood poisoning, urinary tract and kidney infections, and death.

Bacteria are in our food – especially, meat, dairy and poultry products. They can hideout in cuts, sores, nasal passages, under fingernails, and inside root canals or crowns. We can get bacteria from other people, animals, and unclean items.

Bacteria can grow well in a mucous environment. Mucous can be anywhere in the body – digestive tract, sinuses, reproductive organs, lungs and bladder. Drugs and chemicals can contribute to a mucous environment in the body as can foods such as dairy products, meats, poultry, eggs, grains, legumes, and refined sugars. To reduce a mucous environment, eat more fresh greens, fruits, vegetables, and sprouts.

To reduce the risk of bacteria contamination, follow these tips: Be sure to wash your fresh fruits and vegetables well (see above recipe). Always wash your hands before preparing any food. Keep cold foods cold and hot foods hot. Thoroughly cook meats. Add chlorophyll to your diet. Drink plenty of water.

3. **Viruses** are small parasitic microorganisms that come in many forms such as small pox, herpes, HIV/AIDS, Epstein Barr, rabies, and cold viruses. Viruses can hide out in our body for years. They can cause many acute and chronic diseases. Even the residual effects from a previous illness can cause us some health problems. We can contact a virus from other people, animals, or insects. Some viruses are airborne. Viruses also thrive in a mucous environment. *See "Bacteria" above.*

As with parasites and bacteria, viruses can pass through our system and we will not even react to it - if our immune system is strong and our body's environment is clean and healthy.

Foods that can help prevent and treat viral infections are black pepper, garlic, onion, plenty of water, citrus seed extract, and radishes.

4. **Molds / Fungus** – Molds are a multi-cellular fungus. Fungus are microorganisms that are a low form of vegetable life. They can cause superficial and systemic diseases in the body. Many people are allergic to various molds, while others suffer from fungal infections the most common being candida – known as candidiasis.

Candida, that normally live in our body, can become overgrown due to the overuse of antibiotics, oral contraceptives, excess stress or worry, or poor dietary habits and lifestyle. This can cause serious problems in many areas of our body including the blood, tissues, organs, and digestive tract. If antibiotics must be taken, take acidophilus culture to re-establish the healthy flora.

Some symptoms of an overgrowth of candida include,

loss of mental clarity, headaches, recurrent infections, fatigue, food cravings especially for sweets and yeast foods, low immunity, edema, excess mucous, and fungal infections (athletes foot genital yeasts such as vaginitis and jock itch, acne, and ringworm). Serious yeast infections can weaken the immune system leaving it susceptible to other pathogens.

Products that may help fungal infections include 3% food grade hydrogen peroxide (used internally or externally carefully following the directions). Avoid foods that promote candida growth such as concentrated sweeteners, yeast breads, dairy products, eggs, red meats, sweet fruits, and alcoholic beverages. Foods which help this condition are fresh greens, garlic, sprouts, beans, millet, oats, rye, barley, fresh vegetables, sea vegetables, citrus seed extract, garlic, pau d' arco, chlorophyll, and blue-green micro-algae.

1. *List ways you/your family can reduce exposure to and help prevent contamination of the common pathogens. (i.e. wash hands often, bathe regularly, remove pets from the house, cook meat thoroughly)*

DETOXIFICATION

Given the right condition, the body is made to detoxify or eliminate toxins. The problem arises when the immune system is compromised, the organs are stressed or weakened, or the body is polluted to the extent that it cannot perform this process efficiently. This is where we may need to step in and assist the detoxification process.

The first important step in this process is to eliminate the source of the toxicity. For example, if you have amalgam fillings and you are trying to detox from the metals, you would have to have the amalgam fillings removed and replaced with healthier materials.

Symptoms of a disease are the body's way to make us

aware of a problem and cleanse itself. In our society, we are taught to suppress these symptoms in order to make ourselves feel better at the moment. We take medications to stop diarrhea, vomiting, runny noses, or coughing. When we do not allow the natural elimination channels to work and release the toxins from our body, we can retoxify ourselves. Although this can suppress the disease for a time, it may later surface as something even more serious.

The detoxification process varies with individuals. Factors of our body's ability to detoxify include: stress, lifestyle or dietary habits, and exposure to environmental toxins either in our homes or at work. While some people may feel energetic, light, alert, and healthy while detoxifying, others may experience headaches, fatigue, cold or flu like symptoms, or irritability. **Regardless of how you feel during your detoxification process, it is vital that you are consuming plenty of water. Drink 60 % of your weight in ounces of water each day.** *Read Chapter 3: "Consistently stay hydrated" for information regarding the importance of and how to consume water in order to receive the most benefit.*

Always check with your health care practitioner if you are taking medication or have any serious conditions before starting any detoxification program. It is best to consult with your health care practitioner before and during your detox process.

If you are used to eating a high meat, dairy, processed and refined foods diet, a more vegetarian diets consisting of fresh fruits and vegetables, whole grains, and legumes would be a good start in helping the body to cleanse itself. There are also many different types of detoxification programs. **It would be best to consult with your health care practitioner for the program that would be suited for you.** There are many resources available in your local health food stores, herb stores, or alternative health centers to offer more detailed information. Following, is a brief description of some tips and methods that have worked for many people.

REMOVING TOXINS FROM THE BODY

Stimulate the organs of elimination such as the liver, skin, and kidneys. Drugs are hardest to remove from the body because they store in fat cells and various organs especially the liver. The liver is the most highly worked organ in the body. It is the primary organ of detoxification. The liver must transform the toxic substances into a water-soluble compound to be excreted by the kidneys. Milk thistle herb and lemon juice are good cleanses for the liver. For lemon juice, squeeze 1/4 of a lemon in one cup hot water and drink first thing in the morning. When you are detoxing or cleansing, you may go through withdrawals or a healing crisis. Be sure you are drinking plenty of water. (*see suggestions in the "Introduction" on "Things to consider)*

Drink purified water daily, it will help flush the toxins out of the body. *See Chapter 3: "Consistently stay hydrated".* Distilled water can be used for cleansing and removing toxins from the body.

Eat plenty of fiber. It carries bile from the liver and moves it along the intestines so that toxins do not reabsorb back into the body.

Try massage and/or lymph drainage therapy to move toxins from the tissues and the lymph system back into the bloodstream to be eliminated. *See Chapter 9: "Safer, gentler approaches...".*

Exercise consistently to increase blood, oxygen, and lymphatic circulation and to keep your elimination system working efficiently. Exercise increases perspiration, thereby eliminating the toxins through our skin. *See Chapter 7: "Incorporate a regular exercise routine" for types of exercise and the benefits of exercise to stimulate the detoxification process.*

Eat a cleansing diet. Include foods such as whole grains, fresh fruits and vegetables, use cleansing herbs, and drink plenty of water. Avoid foods such as red meat, dairy, fried or fatty foods, sweets and refined products. Try a product specifically for cleansing. They are generally herbal or food based. There are cleanses for the blood, liver, gallbladder, colon (intestines), immune system, lymphatic system, and parasites. *Check with your health care practitioner or your local health food stores for the different types available.*

Have a Colonic / Colema. Colonics are a system whereby water, along with certain nutrients, is used to irrigate and flush out mucous, blockages, toxins, pathogens and old decaying substances from the intestines. Many health care practitioners believe that disease starts in the bowel. If the bowel is not functioning properly, then toxins are not eliminated quickly and end up being reabsorbed back into the blood stream. When we consume foods that are not whole, raw, or contain enough fiber, or if we do not drink plenty of water, we are at risk for serious bowel problems such: cancer of the colon, irritable bowel syndrome, diverticulitis, and other such diseases.

Use homeopathic remedies. They provide nutritional support and stimulate the organ and systems of the body at the cellular level to promote elimination and healing. There are also remedies for detoxification for the lymphatic system, for mucous build up in the body, and for detoxification from metals, chemicals, or pathogens. Homeopathic remedies are safe. Unlike antibiotics that tear down and weaken the immune system, they help to build the body it.

Take a therapeutic bath using mineral crystals, seaweed (dulce, kelp, wakame, kombu), and herbal remedies (ginger, red clover). Many spas offer therapeutic baths, but you can also do them at home. They are relaxing and enjoyable. The skin is the body's largest organ and it can assimilate nutrients quickly and efficiently and detox harmful substances the same way. Be sure to use a dry skin brush before the bath to help open the pores and remove dead skin cells. Fill a tub with very hot water. Meanwhile add the seaweed, herbs, or mineral crystals. You can put them in a tea ball or muslin bag, or you can make a tea and pour it directly into the water. Let the water cool enough to get in and soak from 20-45 minutes.

Fast for a period of time. This can be done in a number of ways such as eating nothing; consuming only water, juices, herbal teas, or broths; or eating certain cleansing foods such as sprouts, grains, fruits, and vegetables – raw or lightly steamed. Fasts can be for one day or for several weeks. The great health and spiritual benefits from a fast have lead many religious and healing organizations to promote some form of fasting.

There are many other benefits of fasting, some of which are overcoming emotional attachments to foods, reducing food allergies, improve sleep and mental focus, and increase clarity of thought and mental awareness. While fasting, be sure to use only good, purified water and foods. Get plenty of rest. Chew your food well.

1. *Depending upon the condition you are concerned about and under the direction of a competent health care practitioner, research and select an appropriate detox program. Follow the program and write down your experiences and feelings throughout the process. Would this program be good to repeat every so often? Is this program one that is specific to a condition to be only completed once?*

2. *Set a goal to continue in the healthy lifestyle change and how you will accomplish it.*

CHAPTER 6

DEVELOP HEALTHIER EATING HABITS

LET YOUR FOOD BE YOUR MEDICINE

Even in the days of superstitions and the beliefs that illnesses were caused by the possession of evil spirits and disfavor of the gods, Hippocrates, in 5th Century B.C., held to the belief that good hygiene, plenty of rest, fresh air, and a good wholesome diet are the natural healing processes of the body. It was he who said, "Let your food be your medicine; Let your medicine be your food". He knew that food contained certain elements that either prevented or healed disease. He was way ahead of his time!

THE HISTORY OF OUR WESTERN DIET

Our country has a "smorgasbord" or "supersize it" attitude when it comes to eating – usually a large quantity and high in cholesterol and saturated fat. We have been lead to believe popular misconceptions such as: "You must eat meat to get enough protein", "You must consume plenty of dairy products to obtain the calcium you need," or "Stay away from starches, such as potatoes, because they will make you fat." Nutrition has long been a topic of debate and there are many different theories that often contradict each other. But, most agree that a healthy diet is based mostly on fruits, vegetables and whole grains.

The rich western diet, commonly referred to as the

Standard American Diet (S.A.D.), focusing on a more meat and dairy based menu, originated approximately 200 years ago. Since then, our society has become increasingly occupied outside of the home, and we have focused more on availability, convenience, and ease of preparation. With these two situations, we began depriving our bodies of the nutritious food it needs. We give up whole grains, replacing then with refined, nutrient deficient products such as white flour, white rice, and sugar. We replaced fresh fruits and vegetables with canned or frozen - or none at all. Generally, our meals not made from scratch; they are often purchased as processed or prepared meals loaded with sodium, preservatives, or other additives with very little nutritional value left.

Such cultures as Native Americans, Asian, and Middle Easterners have enjoyed good health and a high mortality rates without consuming large amounts of animal products and refined, processed foods. However, once they began to eat our western diet, they acquired the same common health problems found in our culture. Many common health problems linked to our western diet are obesity, cancer, heart disease, high blood pressure, osteoporosis, arthritis, diabetes, high cholesterol, asthma, premenstrual syndrome, and menopausal complaints.

IMPORTANCE OF EATING A PLANT BASED DIET

People who eat a plant-based diet generally have less heart disease, obesity, cancer, high cholesterol, stroke, diabetes, and high blood pressure. Their diet usually contains less saturated fat and cholesterol and more nutrition and fiber. Saturated fat is found in animal products such as dairy, eggs, and meat. Vegans consume no cholesterol and very little saturated fat while ova-lacto vegetarian eat a reduced amount compared to the American diet. Protein and other important nutrients are obtained through plants and not animals.

Phytochemicals (plant chemicals) are naturally occurring chemicals in plants that give fruits, vegetables, grains and legumes their medicinal, disease-preventing, health enhancing properties. Containing all of the elements of good nutrition, they consist of vitamins, minerals, fiber, carbohydrates, protein, fat, enzymes, and amino acids. All of which are abundant in the plant kingdom.

The following lists each element of nutrition, along with its role, benefits, and food sources. * *See the food guide pyramids following for servings per day.*

FOOD'S NUTRITIONAL ELEMENTS

AMINO ACIDS
Role – the basic building blocks of proteins that build the muscles, tissues, cells. There are 22 known amino acids. Eight are "essential" - the body cannot make them. Fourteen are "non-essential" - through proper nutrition the body can make them. Consuming a wide variety of vegetable source protein rich foods, we can obtain all the amino acids needed.

Benefits – helps speed wound healing, calms the nervousness system, strengthens the immune and endocrine system, carries oxygen throughout the body, can increase lean tissue to fat tissue body fat ratio which helps in weight management.

Sources – found in protein foods *(see "Protein" below)*

CARBOHYDRATES
Role - the body's fuel for energy. They come from living sources. Carbohydrates release glucose slowly into our system keeping our energy levels even. There are two types of carbohydrates: complex (starches) and simple (sugars). If your diet is too low in complex carbohydrates or too high in sim-

ple carbohydrates, you can increase your risk of diabetes, high blood pressure, heart disease, obesity, tooth decay, anemia, skin problems, kidney disease and cancer. Limit simple carbohydrates, especially those found in refined products. *Caution: Although carbohydrates supply only 4 calories per gram, they can cause weight gain if you live a more sedentary lifestyle because they can be converted into fat and stored by the body. For most people a diet consisting of 50-60% of carbohydrates is ideal.

Benefits – supplies energy to the body, regulates protein and fat metabolism, fights infection, promotes growth of skin and bones, lubricates joints, and helps the body eliminate wastes. They also contain starches and fiber. Starches help to keep blood sugar level by breaking down sugars during digestion.

Sources – simple carbohydrates are found in fruits, honey and refined products containing white flour, white rice, cakes, pastries, breads, cookies, etc. Complex carbohydrates are found in vegetables, grains, and legumes.

ENZYMES

Role – work as catalysts for all activities that occurs in our body. They carry proteins containing nutrients. There are 3 classes of enzymes: metabolic enzymes that run our bodies by healing disease or repairing damage or decay in our organs and tissues; digestive enzymes which digests our food; and food enzymes found in raw food. When we consuming enzyme rich raw foods, we aid food digestion so we are not using the work of our own enzymes for this process.

Cooking food over 118 degrees, destroys enzymes. Processed or junk foods containing chemicals, or caffeine, alcohol, tobacco, chlorine, flouride, or drugs, deplete our body's enzymes. Enzyme deficiency can result in heart disease, cancer, arthritis and pre-mature aging. *Caffeine inhibits an important enzyme (phospho-di-esterage – PDE) that helps in the process of learning and memory development (especially important for those individuals diagnosed with AD/HD or Alzheimer's.

Benefits –digests fat, carbohydrates, and protein. Helps to protect against viral, bacterial, and parasitic infections.

Sources – found in all living things. They are found in all raw food, miso, tofu, tempeh, and soy sauce. Sprouted foods greatly increase enzyme action. Vitamins (especially the B vitamins) and minerals are enzyme helpers.

FATS

Role – are nutritional building blocks for muscles and hormones. They provide insulation in the body. They are a good source of energy and calories, and they make food taste good. Fats are the most concentrated source of food energy, supplying nine calories per gram. Fats can be saturated (solid at room temperature, like shortening, margarine, butter, animal products and palm and coconut oil) or unsaturated (contains important essential fatty acids and are required in the diet).

Essential Fatty Acids (EFA's) are instrumental in energy production, and circulatory system and metabolism function. Deficiency can result in AD/HD, memory loss, autism, learning disabilities, depression, and seizures. If we eat a plant-based diet, we are eating less saturated fat and more essential fatty acids. Two of the most common essential fatty acids are the omega –3 and omega-6 fatty acids. The American (S.A.D) diet is plentiful in the omega-6 fatty acids but are fairly scarce the omega-3 fatty acids.

Limit saturated fats. They are high in calories and usually high in cholesterol. They are mostly found in animal products. Eat 10-20% of your calories from fat (the average diet is about 42%! To reduce this percent greatly reduce or eliminate meat and dairy).

Trans-fatty acids are made by processing oils through

hydrogen - a procedure called hydrogenation. This procedure destroys the vitamin E and changes the physical form of the oil and the way the body metabolizes these fats. The fats now become saturated and very toxic. They are in margarine, shortening, regular vegetable oils found in the grocery store and in many processed and refined foods. Be sure to buy cold-pressed or expeller-pressed oils. Trans-fatty acids can cause problems with digestion, pregnancy, the liver, the heart, immune system function, obesity, diabetes, and cancer.
Benefits – provides a feeling of satiety. EFA's reduce the risk of heart disease, prevent dryness of the skin and hair, improve AD/HD symptoms, help in the absorption of vitamins, reduces PMS symptoms, aide in digestion, lower cholesterol, improve liver function, help with weight loss, and help in brain and emotional development.
Sources – omega-3's include flax and evening primrose oil, canola oil, wheat germ oil, walnuts and seafood. Omega-6's include olive oil, nuts and seeds along with their oils, bananas, avocados, butter, corn, beans, and soybeans.

FIBER
Role - is the indigestible part of the plant. It comes in two forms: insoluble and soluble. Insoluble fiber is found in whole grains, cereals, wheat bran and many fruits and vegetables. Soluble fiber is found in oats, dried beans, apples and citrus fruits. Eat about 35 grams of fiber per day (the average American only eats about 13 grams per day!)
Benefits – keeps the intestines properly functioning and eliminating by absorbing water and speeding up transit time to prevent constipation. It binds to fat and carries it out of the body keeping it from being absorbed into the system thereby preventing weight gain and reducing cholesterol. It can bind up toxins such as mercury, arsenic or lead in the intestines and removes them through elimination. It prevents diverticulosis, cancer, heart disease, stroke, ulcers and gastrointestinal prob-

lems. It keeps blood sugar and energy levels even. It improves digestion and fills you up so you are less hungry.

Sources - the skin of fruits or vegetables and the coverings on the grains such as bran. Also tomato and vegetable juices contain fiber. Beans, vegetables, fruits, cereal grains and whole grains are all great sources of fiber. There are also many fiber supplements available in pill and powder form. The best way to get your fiber is through your diet.

MINERALS

Role – help to build the body. They also help the body use vitamins. All of the activities in our body require minerals. They help to maintain the cellular fluid balance to form bone and blood cells, regulate all muscle and organ activity, and help to provide nerve signaling responses throughout the body.

Because minerals are primarily stored in bone and muscle tissue, there is a risk of toxicity if large amounts are consumed through supplementation. Mineral imbalances can cause conditions such as depression, suicidal tendencies, nervousness, forgetfulness and fatigue. Imbalances can also cause physical conditions such as: muscle spasms, cramps, insomnia, cancer, skin or hair problems, frequent illnesses, arthritis, and osteoporosis.

We obtain minerals through the plants we eat. Plants do not manufacture minerals, they absorb them from the soil they grow in and then we eat the plants.

Benefits – build the body, help to release emotional blocks, and have in many therapeutic uses.

Sources – dried fruits, plant, and animal foods.

PROTEIN

Role – required for production of hormones, enzymes, tissues, and antibodies. It is a source of energy and important for growth and development. When we eat protein our body breaks it down into the amino acids that it is composed of. The amino acids, in return, make the protein required to build the body – i.e. muscle.

There are two classes of protein, complete and incomplete. Complete protein contains all of the essential amino acids. They are found in all animal products. Incomplete protein contains some of the amino acids needed by the body. They are found in grains, vegetables and legumes. If you are eating a vegan diet, it is important to eat a variety of foods to ensure you are getting complete protein.

You may combine certain foods to be sure you are getting enough complete protein such as: beans with brown rice, corn, seeds, nuts or wheat, or brown rice with seeds, wheat, or nuts.

A high protein diet, especially protein from animal products, has been linked to diseases such as arthritis and osteoporosis. The animal protein causes the blood to become acidic and dissolves the calcium from the bones. The calcium is then excreted through the urine. It can also cause immune system related diseases. The molecules are large and hard to digest and they plug up the lymphatic system.

The average American diet contains about 100 grams of protein per day. We only need about 35-50 grams. Protein supplies 4 calories per gram. To estimate the daily amount of grams of protein needed, take your ideal weight and divide by 2.75.

Benefits – curbs the appetite while promoting satiety after a meal, builds muscles that burn up calories, increases energy,

Sources – soy foods contain the essential amino acids such as tofu, soymilk, soy cheese, soy flour and tempeh; lean meats and fish; beans, and grains. Avoid proteins high in fat, cholesterol, and calories.

VITAMINS

Role –help to control the flow of minerals through the body and help metabolize and utilize those minerals. They work together with enzymes to release energy from digested food, and regulate the chemical activities that occur in the body. There are two types of vitamins: fat-soluble and water-soluble. Fat-soluble vitamins are A, D, E and K. They are found in the fatty portions of food and can store in the body's fatty tissues and liver. They are excreted in the intestines and are either reabsorbed back into the body or are excreted through the feces. Too high of an intake can result in toxicity. Water-soluble vitamins are C and the B's. They are not stored in the body so they must be consumed every day. They are excreted through the urine and usually do not reach such toxic levels as can fat-soluble vitamins.

Although some may argue that "the body doesn't know the difference between food based or synthetic vitamins, so it doesn't matter what form you take", we have found that synthetic vitamins can be very toxic. – especially to the liver. If a vitamin reads "high-potency" it will be synthetic.

Benefits – help to prevent and heal disease, help the body to absorb and assimilate minerals, and prevent health problems related to deficiency.

Sources – fat-soluble vitamins are found in the fats in foods. Water-soluble vitamins are found in legumes, grains, fruits, vegetables, meat and dairy foods.

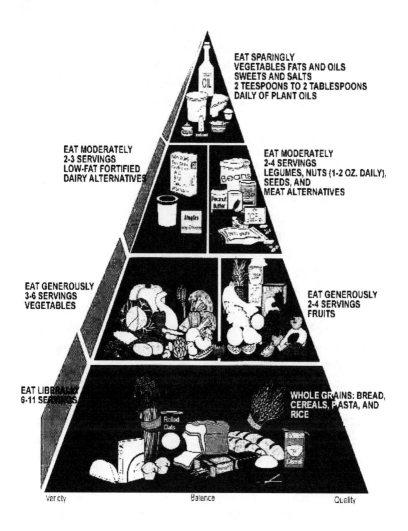

EAT SPARINGLY
VEGETABLES FATS AND OILS
SWEETS AND SALTS
2 TEESPOONS TO 2 TABLESPOONS
DAILY OF PLANT OILS

EAT MODERATELY
2-3 SERVINGS
LOW-FAT FORTIFIED
DAIRY ALTERNATIVES

EAT MODERATELY
2-4 SERVINGS
LEGUMES, NUTS (1-2 OZ. DAILY),
SEEDS, AND
MEAT ALTERNATIVES

EAT GENEROUSLY
3-6 SERVINGS
VEGETABLES

EAT GENEROUSLY
2-4 SERVINGS
FRUITS

EAT LIBERALLY
6-11 SERVINGS

WHOLE GRAINS: BREAD,
CEREALS, PASTA, AND
RICE

Variety   Balance   Quality

TIPS TO GETTING THE MOST NUTRITION FROM FOOD

Many things can influence the nutritional value of our food. Although some of the foods we eat are becoming depleted in nutrients due to unfertile soil; laced with harmful chemicals, herbicides and pesticides; or are picked before maturity, there are things we can do at home to help bring up the nutritional content of our food.

1. Like humans, foods have energy. When foods are refrigerated, they have a lower energy level. By warming, tossing, stirring or adding fresh herbs and spices we can raise their energy level making them more nutritious.

2. Focus on the food you are eating – the taste, texture, aroma, enjoyment, and how the food is benefiting you. Do not watch T.V., read, or other activities. It can inhibit your digestion and assimilation of important nutrients.

3. When preparing food, your own energy and emotions can affect the foods quality. Try not to prepare food when you are angry or upset. The foods energy will be higher if you feel love and happiness for the people you are serving and for the food itself. This is one reason why the food in restaurants, especially fast food establishments, are not as nutritious as what you would prepare at home. Seldom the food is prepared with love.

4. Always wash your fresh foods and vegetables before eating them with a diluted solution of food grade hydrogen peroxide and water. About 1/4 cup per sink full of water. This will help to remove any pesticides or other chemicals or substances found on them.

5. Buy organically grown products when possible for two reasons. One, they are free from harmful chemicals, and two, they have a higher energy level due to the care and concern of the people who produce them.

6. Canned foods have a low nutritional value and through the heating process destroys the enzymes. It has no oxygen and little or no energy. Try to eat fresh foods when possible.

7. Frozen fruits and vegetables are destroyed at a cellular level lowering the energy level. Choose fresh foods when possible.

8. If you can't always have fresh foods, then dried foods would be the next choice. Dry your own fresh food instead of canning or freezing. It contains more nutrients, takes up less space, stores easier (just stack on a shelf) and is cheaper to prepare and store.

9. Do not cook food in a microwave. It completely destroys the enzymes and can change the chemical composition of the food. Foods will have little or no energy level.

10. Try to eat at least 50% of all of your foods raw. 60-70% would be even better. You will get more nutrients, energy and enzymes.

11. When you do cook your vegetables, lightly steam or quickly stir-fry them. It will help to retain more nutrients as compared to boiling or frying.

12. Eat fruits either in the morning, during a snack time or at least 20 minutes before a meal. Fruits digest the fastest. If they do not leave the stomach and small intestines quickly enough, (because they are mixed with other foods that take a lot longer time to digest) the fruits will ferment. This can cause digestive problems and prevents weight loss.

13. Grow your own food. Even if you only have a small patio, you can grow quite a bit. The food will be healthier because you can pick it ripe, grow it organically, and grow it with love.

14. Try to buy tree-ripened or vine-ripened fruits or vegetables. When fruits or vegetables are picked too green, many of the nutrients are missing. During the ripening process the plant sends sugar along with the nutrients directly to the fruit or vegetable just a few days before it is ready to be picked. That's when it's energy level and nutritional value is the highest.

15. Although it is not imperative that you always do proper food combining, you can compliment your meals and increase then nutritional values: i.e. eat beans with corn or rice to make a complete protein; blend tofu into your favorite fruit drink for added calcium and protein; add fresh herbs to your salad or cooked casserole dish for extra enzymes nutrients and energy; or add a tablespoon of molasses to your bowl of granola for an extra boost of iron. *As long as you eat a mixture of proteins throughout the day, you will get enough of the essential amino acids.

16. Throw out all of your hydrogenated oil products such as shortening, margarine, cooking oils and products made with this oil. Replace them with cold-pressed or expeller-pressed vegetable oils.

CHANGING OUR LIFESTYLE

We must make our food choices dependent on a healthy lifestyle, not on family traditions, geographic locations, convenience, habits, social atmosphere, or our "microscopic" taste buds. We have trained ourselves over the years to acquire tastes for certain types of foods. Among them are foods high in sugar and fat. We can retrain our taste buds to enjoy fresh, whole foods equally as much. It is important to try to eat at least 50% of our foods raw. This means more fresh fruits and vegetables. While diet is very important to our state of health, there are other things that can impact it. Not only do we need to eat proper foods, but add to our environment moderate exercise, adequate sunshine, clean air and water, a positive attitude, and comfortable surroundings. Food can be fun, rewarding, comforting, enjoyable, and delicious.

1. *List all of the foods you have eaten in a 24-hour period.*

2. *Are at least 50% of the foods raw?*

3. *List ways you can add more raw foods to you/your family's diet. (i.e. try different salad dressings and salads, eat fresh fruit for breakfast, precut fresh raw vegetables and fruits for snacks, put them on sandwiches, roll them up into burritos,, etc. * "See I Love to Eat Vegetarian!" cookbook, and other "A New Hope for Health" series cookbooks)*

4. *List ways you can make mealtime a quiet, peaceful, uninterrupted environment whereby me/my family can enjoy the time and gain the most benefit from our food?(i.e. take the phone off the hook, try to get as many people together at mealtime as possible, have a set time that meals will be served, turn off the T.V., etc)*

6. *If you are used to cooking in a microwave, what other options do I have that would still be as quick and efficient? (i.e. small toaster oven for reheating, crock pot that can be started quickly in the morning, learn to stir-fry or steam, or use the "Time Bake" on the oven, etc)*

CHAPTER 7

INCORPORATE A REGULAR EXERCISE ROUTINE

MOVE IT AND LOSE IT!

We live in an area that borders state and national parks. Because the winters are mild, we enjoy many outdoor activities. Besides the typical hiking, biking, and golfing, there are 5K, 10K, half marathon, and marathon foot races held throughout the year. It is fun to see people of all ages enjoying the activities. I run most of the races, and I am amazed and impressed when I see people 20 years older than I am passing me right up!   It's great to see people in their 70's and 80's still active and working hard to take good care of themselves.

We're never too young or old for some form of exercise. At any age we can receive health benefits and add years to our life. You have probably heard sayings like "Use it or lose it" or "If you rest you'll rust". Well, they are true. Exercise is one of the best ways to improve your health, lose weight, reduce stress, and gives you an overall sense of well being.

For many though, exercise is a dirty word and there is nothing worse than having to do something you really dread. Why do some people choose not to exercise? Read on!

1. "I just don't have the time"
2. "It's too cold / hot outside"
3. "It hurts"
4. "It's faster to drive"

5. "I'm just too tired"
6. "I'm too out of shape"
7. "I don't feel well"
8. "It's too much effort"
9. "I don't like exercising"
10. "I'm too old"
11. "I'll embarrass my self"
12. "I'll start tomorrow..."

Maybe you have heard or even used some of these reasons. You can probably think of more. Once you understand some of the benefits of exercise and some tips for exercising, you may be more motivated to find some form of activity that you enjoy.

1.   *Pretend someone is telling you one of these reasons. Write down what your response or solution would be if you were trying to convince him/her of the need for exercise.*

2.   *Can this solution work for you, too? If so, how?*

BENEFITS OF EXERCISING

1. **Reduces stress.** Exercising increases our oxygen intake thereby activating important chemicals in the brain such as: endorphins, adrenaline, serotonin, and dopamine that produce feelings of pleasure and give you that "natural high". Therefore, exercise can reduce depression and anxiety, often without the use of drugs. It also provides better relaxation, sleep, and sexual responses. It helps to improve our mood. It is a good way to get the "attitude adjustment" we sometimes need.

Exercise can clear our mind and improve mental vigor, creativity, and imagination. It allows us the time to sort things out in our mind helping us to solve problems or come up with new ideas. It helps us handle mental challenges better. Our self-esteem and confidence are lifted because we look and feel better. We increase self-mastery, discipline, enthusiasm, and optimism. Developing these qualities helps us to adhere to any new lifestyle changes.

Yoga and Tai'Chi exercises are great relaxation exercises.

2. Detoxifies the body. Our lymphatic system ("sewer system") accumulates toxins and garbage in our system and flushes it out through our blood stream and kidneys. Sometimes it becomes sluggish or even blocked, often by large protein molecules from consuming too many animal products. When this happens we can become sick. Exercise stimulates the lymphatic system helping it release toxins through our skin (by perspiration) and through our eliminatory organs.

Best exercises are aerobic type activities such as running, race walking, swimming, or aerobic classes, and jumping on a jogger tramp or trampoline.

3. Slows down the aging process. Exercise can add quality years to our life. It is beneficial to the cardiovascular system, which is the main cause for mortality in older adults. The heart becomes stronger and larger so less effort is needed to pump the blood. It circulates more blood per beat resulting in a lower resting heart rate. For the maximum benefit, elevate the heart rate for at least 20 minutes (*be sure you can still carry on a conversation without gasping for air*). It helps to reduce blood pressure by keeping the blood vessels more elastic and clear of fat. This allows for better circulation.

Exercise helps our skin retain a more youthful appearance by releasing toxins and excess salt through perspiration. Perspiration contains chemicals that keep our skin soft and elastic. It also increases the circulation needed to carry oxygen and nutrients to our cells that keeps us youthful and alert. *Strength training and aerobic exercise are great exercises to help slow down the aging process.*

4. Controls weight. If you diet to lose weight without exercising, you will lose about 25% of your lean body mass. We want to keep all of the lean body mass (muscle, tissue, etc) we can and lose only the fat. Exercise burns calories by raising our metabolic rate. *It takes 20 minutes or more of aerobic exercise to start burning fat.* The longer you work out (past the 20 minutes) the more fat and calories you burn. The good news is that we can continue to burn calories for up to 24 hours <u>after</u> the activity. When we burn calories we decrease our body fat.

If you decide to have your body fat analyzed, a guide to consider is: women should be in the 18-24% range with 32% on the edge of obesity, and men should be in the 12-17% range with 23% on the edge of obesity. If you are 20% or more over your ideal weight, you are considered obese. *See the height and weight char at the end of this chapter.*

Aerobic activity is best for weight loss, although strength training can burn fat too.

5. Improves muscle tone and flexibility, and builds bone mass. After the age of 30 we start to loses bone mass. Weight bearing type exercises helps bones become denser and stronger which helps prevent and treat such conditions as osteoporosis and osteoarthritis. When our skeletal system is strong there is less chance of falling or injury. Exercise helps us to stay flexible and build muscle mass thereby reducing pain and stiffness that comes from a more sedentary lifestyle. Good muscle tone keeps our organs and bones in their proper place. *Weight bearing exercises include free weights, weight*

*machines, elastic bands or cords, or whatever you have at
home – cans, bottles filled with water, etc)*

A major complaint in our society is back pain. Many of
us have poor posture, are over weight, live a more sedentary
lifestyle, eat an unhealthy diet and, are under a great deal of
stress. Any of which can lead to back problems. Generally,
back pain comes from muscle tension and not from the bones
themselves. Exercises that focus on flexibility and strengthening the abdomen and back may help to prevent many back
problems.

*Stretching and weight bearing exercises help most with
flexibility and strength, and crunches and abdomen work-
outs tone the abdomen thereby strengthening the back.*

6. **Improves overall health.** Exercise raises our energy
level by increasing oxygen and blood circulation, and keeping muscles stronger so it takes less effort for any activity. We
speed up our metabolism and burn fat which also increases
energy. We can also tolerate and adapt to cold and heat more
easily.

Our appetite improves. We have the ability to eat more
and not gain weight. Provided we eat healthy, this permits a
greater intake of all nutrients. After we have exercised for 1/2
hour our appetite can decrease. This can help keep us from
snacking and eating the wrong things.

It has been shown to improve conditions such as: allergies, high blood pressure, elevated cholesterol, diabetes, obesity, cancer, cardiovascular, Parkinson's, Alzheimer's, M.S.,
gastrointestinal problems, bowel function, insomnia, fatigue,
and stroke. We can also reduce the amount of colds or flu.

7. **Saves money.** There are less health problems for people that stay physically active because we lower our risk factors for serious conditions, accidents, and illnesses. We have
less medical expenses, because there are less trips to the doc-

tor's office or hospital. People who exercise regularly are less likely to smoke, drink, take drugs, or involve themselves in expensive unhealthy habits. Weight loss drugs and programs are very expensive-exercise is cheap. Once a person is off the drug or program, the weight usually returns within a year or so because necessary lifestyle changes were not made that originally caused the weight gain.

EXERCISE TIPS

1. To gain the maximum cardiovascular benefit and burn the greatest number of calories, choose exercises that are continuous or uninterrupted like: walking, running, cycling, hiking, endurance exercise machines, swimming, rowing machines, dancing, treadmill, stair steppers, etc.

2. Exercise helps you to build lean body mass and decrease body fat. In order to burn fat you must exercise aerobically for **at least 20 minutes**. Anytime after 20 minutes you will continue to burn fat and calories. Set your goal for about 45 minutes a day, 3-4 times a week.

3. Always warm up before exercising to prevent injury and cool down after a workout using stretching exercises to prevent injury or sore muscles. Breathe deeply while stretching. It helps your muscles to relax and lowers your blood pressure.

4. When stretching, never bounce the stretch because you may tear muscle fibers or tendons. Hold each stretch for at least 10 seconds. You should feel tension, but not any pain.

5. Drink water before, during, and after exercising. You should drink 24 ounces of water for every one hour of continuous activity where you are perspiring or elevating your heart rate. Drinking water also helps to prevent injury and sore

muscles.

6. Wait a couple of hours after eating to exercise vigor-
ously. You body is using your blood to help in the digestive
process and you need it in your muscles when exercising.

7. Start off slow when beginning a new exercise program. Some people are too ambitious at first and either injure
themselves or become too tired or exhausted to continue.

8. Consider these 4 things when choosing an exercise:
a. Choice of activity – Will it help me accomplish my
goal? (Health benefits, weight loss, interests, etc)
b. Frequency – How often can I exercise? (4 times a
week? On Saturdays? Be sure to schedule one day a week to
rest)
c. Intensity – How hard should I work out? What is my
target heart rate? What is my energy level?
d. Duration – How long can each exercise period be? (45
minutes per day? An hour? etc)

9. Choose aerobic exercise if you wish to build
endurance, elevate your heart rate for an extended period of
time, reduce body fat, reduce cholesterol, strengthen bones and
spine, lower your risk of heart attacks, strokes diabetes, cancer, and give yourself an overall feeling of well-being. For
maximum benefit: 45 minutes 3-4 times per week.

10. Choose strength training exercises if you wish to
maintain or improve upper body strength, build muscle
strength, burn fat, maintain or improve bone density, improve
digestion, lower cholesterol, or reverse the effects of aging.
Maximum benefit is 10-20 minutes 2-3 times per week.

11. Choose flexibility (stretching) training if you wish to

develop a wider range of motion, relax, lower blood pressure, reduce stress, strengthen or relax your back, prevent injuries, prevent muscle cramps or stiffness, or improve your balance, strength or flexibility. It is important to stretch after any kind of workout. For maximum benefit, stretch 10-15 minutes for 3 times a week.

EXERCISE CAUTIONS

1. Check with your health care practitioner as to the type and amount of exercise you choose, especially if you have any health conditions or are on medication.

2. Avoid using diuretics such as drugs, caffeine, and alcohol. They can reduce your body's ability to regulate internal temperature (you can over heat), and electrolyte balance (lose valuable minerals).

3. Using beta-blockers (drugs used for hypertension) may keep you from reaching your desired heart rate because they slow down your heart rate and blood pressure.

4. Over the counter pills, cold remedies, or nicotine can increase or decrease heart rate and blood pressure.

5. When strenuously exercising where you are perspiring heavily, be sure to drink a good sports drink to help replace the lost electrolytes. This helps to avoid dehydration, fatigue, and muscle problems. Also be sure you are still drinking at least 60% of your body weight in water each day.

1.   *List any of the reasons you have used to avoid exercising and how you can overcome them. (i.e. I just don't have the time – so I will get up 1/2 hour earlier each day of the week)*

2.   List any physical activities you enjoy doing and what
     options are available to you. (i.e. mountains to hike, a
     weight gym to attend)

3.   Write down the time available during the day or week
     for exercising and how long each exercise period can be.
     (i.e. 5 days a week before dinner for one hour)

4.   Write down how you can reach your goal for increasing
     your physical activity. (i.e. sign up for swimming classes,
     plan weekly hikes, walk with a friend)

PHYSICAL FITNESS CALCULATIONS

Below are formulas and charts used to find your **target
heart rate, estimating caloric requirements, estimating number of grams of fat per day, average calories burned per hour,
and target body weight** if you would like to make your own
calculations. Many weight gyms, weight programs, or health
clubs can figure these and your body fat content for you.
Body fat content: Women should be in the 17-24% range with
32% on the edge of obesity, and men should be in the 12-
17% range with 23% on the edge of obesity.

1. Target Heart Rate

220 – (your age)= _____(maximum heart rate)

_____(maximum heart rate) X .65 = _____(fat burn-
ing level)

_____(maximum heart rate) X . 80 = _____(aerobic
level)

Depending on your fitness level (it can change), you can

adjust your target heart rate by multiplying your maximum heart rate by the percentage level you feel you qualify for. Work in that target heart rate until your condition changes. Then...

_____(maximum heart rate) X 40-60% for the deconditioned

X 50-70% for the average exerciser

X 60-80% for the more fit

To find if you are in your target heart rate:
Count your heartbeats for 10 seconds and then multiply that by 6 to get the beats per minute.

2. Estimating Daily Caloric Requirements

Take your **target** (ideal) weight and multiply it by:
10% for light activity
15% for moderate activity
20% for heavy activity

Then, subtract 100 calories for age 35-44
200 calories for age 45-54
300 calories for age 55-64
400 calories for age 65 and up

Example: Target weight is 125 pounds. Activity is moderate.

125 X 15 = 1875 calories per day

If you are 45 then it would be 1875 − 200 = 1675 calories per day

This is how many calories you would need to consume to arrive at your target weight depending on your activity level you entered.

    * You should not consume less than 1200 calories per day.

3. Estimating Number of Grams of Fat Per Day

To stay healthy or to maintain or lose weight we should consume between 10-20% calories from fat each day. To figure this, take your **daily caloric requirement** (figured above) and multiply it by the percentage of fat. (15 or 20)
Then, divide calories from fat by 9 (fat calories per gram) to give you the number of grams of fat per day.

    Example: 1675 cal. per day X 20% (cal. from fat) = 335 cal. from fat
    335 cal. from fat / 9 = 37 grams of fat per day

4. Average Calories Burned Per Hour of Activity

The averages below (AHA source) gives you an idea of the number of calories burned through continuous exercise in the various areas. *You need to burn 3,500 calories just to lose 1 pound of fat!* Figure your caloric requirement using the formula (step 2.)

Activity	Calories burned per hr.
Basketball	360

Bicycling (6 mph)	240
Bicycling (12 mph)	410
Jogging (5.5 mph)	740
Jogging (7 mph)	920
Jumping Rope	750
Running in place	650
Running (10 mph)	1,280
Skiing (cross-country)	700
Swimming (25 yds/min)	275
Swimming (50 yds/min)	500
Tennis (singles)	400
Walking (2 mph)	240
Walking (4 mph)	440
Weight Training	300
Wrestling	540

5. Waist-to-hip ratio

It is important to figure your waist-to-hip ratio. If your value is greater than 1.0, it means that the measurement of your hips is larger than the measurement of your waist. If so, you could be at risk for more serious health conditions because you are carrying too much fat around the abdomen area and vital organs. Keep your values under 0.85 for women and 0.95 for men. Use the following formula.

Stand relaxed, and measure around your waist. Don't pull in your stomach. Then measure around the largest part of your hips. Divide your waist measurement by your hip measurement. This will give you your waist-to-hip ratio.

Example: Waist measurement = 32 in., Hip measurement = 34 in. 32 / 34 = .94

HEIGHT & WEIGHT TABLES

MEN

Height Feet/Inches	Small Frame	Medium Frame	Large Frame
5'2"	128-134	131-141	138-150
5'3"	130-136	133-143	140-153
5'4"	132-138	135-145	142-156
5'5"	134-140	137-148	144-160
5'6"	136-142	139-151	146-164
5'7"	138-145	142-154	149-168
5'8"	140-148	145-157	152-172
5'9"	142-151	148-160	155-176
5'10"	144-154	151-163	158-180
5'11"	146-157	154-166	161-184
6'0"	149-160	157-170	164-188
6'1"	152-164	160-174	168-192
6'2"	155-168	164-178	172-197
6'3"	158-172	167-182	176-202
6'4"	162-176	171-187	181-202

Weights at ages 25-59 based on lowest mortality.
Weight in pounds according to frame (indoor
clothing weighing 5 lbs.; shoes with 1" heels

WOMEN

Height Feet/Inches	Small Frame	Medium Frame	Large Frame
4'10"	102-111	109-121	118-131
4'11"	103-113	111-123	120-134
5'0"	104-115	113-126	122-137
5'1"	106-118	115-129	125-140
5'2"	108-121	118-132	126-143
5'3"	111-124	121-135	131-147
5'4"	114-127	124-138	134-151
5'5"	117-130	127-141	137-155
5'6"	120-133	130-144	140-159
5'7"	123-166	133-147	143-163
5'8"	126-139	136-150	146-167
5'9"	129-142	139-153	149-170
5'10"	132-145	142-156	152-173
5'11"	135-148	145-159	155-176
6'0"	138-151	148-162	158-179

Weights at ages 25-59 based on lowest mortality.
Weight in pounds according to frame (indoor
clothing weighing 3 lbs.; shoes with 1" heels

CHAPTER 8

ACHIEVE AND MAINTAIN IDEAL WEIGHT

FREE TO A GOOD HOME-

THOSE UNWANTED POUNDS!

In the early 1990's, I was beginning to put on a few pounds. I was exercising daily and trying to eat healthy (lots of fruits and vegetables from our garden, and whole grains – some meat and dairy). By the end of 3 years I had gained 15 pounds. I was becoming frustrated not knowing what else to do. I decided to have a blood test done to see if there were any physical problems. The doctor informed me that my thyroid was functioning too low. He said that I was to come back in a few months to have it checked again, and that if it were any lower, I would need to go on thyroid medication.

I remembered back when I had taken my son off dairy products because of the reoccurring tonsillitis, and then learning about all of the childhood illnesses it had been linked to. I decided to read and study all that I could on thyroid, weight problems, etc. – starting with meat and dairy. I read how dairy products can cause many glandular problems, especially thyroid. I also read how substances (hormones, preservatives, etc.) put in animal products can also cause weight problems. Although we ate a fairly balanced diet, I was eating either some kind of meat or dairy practically every day. I decided to put this new knowledge to the test.

I went through all of my recipes looking for ways to

modify them or use dairy and meat substitutions. I ordered two vegetarian magazines. I bought a few vegetarian cookbooks. Then, I went through my pantry and threw everything away that contained any animal products, food additives, preservatives, and processed foods. It was pretty bare when I was through. I bought a new blender and wheat grinder and loaded up on whole grains such as wheat, kamut, spelt, rice, corn, etc.

It was not easy changing how I cooked and what my family had been used to eating, but it was fun seeing how colorful, tasty, and healthier our new dishes were. I did not change my exercise program – only improved the foods we were eating. After about 5 months, the 15 pounds had vanished. I waited 2 years before going back to the doctor (I wanted to be sure to give my body plenty of time to heal itself and make permanent changes). I then had another blood test. My thyroid was normal! The doctor was definitely surprised – especially when I told him how I healed it myself! Little did I know that this change in my diet would bring other health benefits I had never even thought of. No more allergy attacks in the spring and fall! What a welcomed relief!

There are hundreds of diets out there today promoted by our culture as a way to lose weight and keep it off. We are constantly bombarded with the "new diet that really works!" on T.V., in magazines, on the radio, in the doctor's office, and from our neighbors. If these diets are so successful, then why are approximately 60-70% of Americans still over weight? Most of these people have tried numerous diets throughout their lives and are still struggling to either lose weight or keep off the weight they have lost. **There is no magic bullet when it comes to losing weight and keeping it off!**

Many people come to us seeking advice on how to lose weight. Their reasons vary from improving their looks, preventing or reversing illnesses, improving overall health and energy, dealing with concerns from loved ones, or depression from all of the past weight loss failures.

What is the reason(s) you/someone you know wishes to shed those unwanted pounds?

COMMON BARRIERS TO LOSING WEIGHT

Just as there are barriers that can prevent us from being healthy, there are barriers that can prevent us from losing weight. Even though there can be a lot at stake from being overweight, there are some who justify remaining that way. Below are some common barriers we often hear.

1. "Big bones and over weight runs in my family"
2. "I don't want to be bothered by men/women"
3. "I'm happy just the way I am"
4. "It's just part of getting older"
5. "I don't have the willpower"
6. "It's too hard"
7. "I have to eat out a lot"
8. "My family refuses to eat this way, so it's hard to do this alone"
9. "I'd rather just take a drug or have a surgery"
10. "I'll just gain the weight back"

Of course, there are other factors to consider regarding weight loss such as: stress, physical or health conditions, or medications. But, even these factors can be improved by following the suggestions in this chapter.

1. *Can you think of any other barriers that people use?*

2. *Write down the barriers you/someone you know have used or are presently using.*

3. *Are any of these barriers keeping you/someone you*

know from obtaining ideal weight? If yes, would you/someone you know like to overcome them?

4. *What can you do overcome these barriers? (i.e. learn to eat healthier when eating out, avoid the self-limiting beliefs and change the negative self-talk to positive, set goals and stick to them no matter if you have support or not)*

THINGS TO CONSIDER

1. Simple carbohydrates. When we consume too many simple carbohydrates such as: refined products (sugar, white flour, white rice, pastries, too many fruits, etc.), we can weaken our kidneys and adrenal glands causing us to feel tired. When we feel tired, we are not motivated to get up and exercise, fix healthy meals, arise early in the morning, or do those things that would encourage weight loss. Eating more complex carbohydrates (vegetables, fruits, whole grains, beans, legumes) can increase our energy level. The more energetic we feel, the more we are willing to exercise and eat healthy. Also, simple carbohydrates absorb more calories in the intestines than do complex carbohydrates. They also raise our insulin levels. Insulin can cause our fat cells to accumulate fat and then prevents them from releasing it.

2. Artificial Sweeteners. These are chemicals found in diet products and have been known to contribute to weight gain. Aspartame (Nutrasweet, equal, Spoonfuletc.) is a chemical that can cross the blood brain barrier reaching the hypothalamus, thereby causing this gland to send out messages that we are hungry – so we snack. These products usually contain a great deal of salt, phosphates, and other products that can lead to other health problems.

3. Alcohol. It can raise our insulin levels by increasing the absorption of sugar from the intestines. This causes fat cells to accumulate fat, and then prevents the fat from being burned. So, if your eating a high fat diet and consuming alcohol, you can gain weight. Alcohol usually contains a lot of sugar and 210 calories per ounce.

4. **Dieting.** This is not a healthy way to lose weight. When we deprive ourselves of food it can harm us mentally (our brain needs fuel to function), physically (we need nutrients to stay healthy), and emotionally (we can become depressed feeling we are deprived or sacrificing simple pleasures). We are made to eat and to enjoy food in all of its varieties. Diets to lose weight often are not balanced, and can lead to serious health problems.

High protein diets can place a strain on the kidneys and liver and can be high in cholesterol and saturated fat. This kind of eating habit has been related to cancer, heart disease, high cholesterol, digestive problems (due to lack of fiber), and diabetes.

Diets that eliminate complex carbohydrates (vegetables, fruits, whole grains, beans legumes, etc.) also eliminate many valuable vitamins and minerals our bodies need to stay healthy and energetic. Carbohydrates are our hunger drive – our basic source of fuel for energy. Carbohydrates will satisfy your body's needs so you will automatically eat less as time goes on.

Complex carbohydrates also provide fiber that binds with fat (which goes into our tissues) and cholesterol (which goes into our blood) and removes them from the body before it can be reabsorbed back into our system. Fiber also binds with water and increases the volume of food in the stomach. This helps you to feel satisfied so you take in fewer calories. Fiber helps to reduce our risk of certain cancers and digestive problems, lowers cholesterol, and helps us to lose weight.

When we deprive ourselves of food, (skipping meals,

not eating enough calories, etc.) our body goes into a "famine" mode. This saves our lives in times of scarcity of food. In order to do that, the metabolism slows down causing you to burn fewer calories. You also lose considerable muscle mass along with the fat. If you gain the weight back it is usually all fat, so you end up with more fat than muscle than you had originally.

5. **Animal Products.** The growth hormones and steroids given to animals have possibly been linked to chemical and hormonal imbalances in humans. These kinds of imbalances could contribute to weight gain. Animal products are high in saturated fat and cholesterol which has also been linked to weight gain. Animal products can plug up our lymphatic system. A plugged lymphatic system not only can cause disease but edema, cellulite, and slow circulation.

6. **Caffeine.** For some people caffeine can cause such an acidic environment in their body that the body tries to retain water to neutralize it. It also causes the body to retain water because it is a diuretic and causes dehydration. Water retention causes weight gain. *See "Caffeine" in Chapter 9: "Avoid exposure to toxic chemicals".*

7. **Estrogen Replacement Therapy (ERT).** Because of its synthetic forms, they have been known to contribute to weight gain. Try a more natural approach if possible (Dong Quai, wild yam, etc). Birth control pills and hormones such as progesterone can also contribute to weight gain.

8. **Thyroid.** This gland regulates our metabolism (the amount of calories burned in a specific time). It can also accumulate many toxins. If it is sluggish, your metabolism slows down causing you to gain weight. You can perform a simple test at home to see if your thyroid gland is functioning prop-

erly. Take your temperature in the morning before rising. If it is below 97.6, your thyroid is not working efficiently. If it is low, there are things you can do to boost your metabolism.

a. **Exercise** helps to remove toxins from lungs, perspiration and lymphatic system . Yoga exercises can actually stimulate the thyroid. * *See Chapter 7: "Incorporate a regular exercise routine" for more information regarding weight loss.*

b. **Dairy products** have been associated with glandular problems, especially the thyroid, mainly because of the products they contain such as casein and antibiotics. Dairy products are very mucous forming. The mucous can settle in many different areas of the body causing a hardship and sluggishness in our organs, glands, intestinal tract, and various other areas.

c. **Hydrogenated and brominated oils** have been linked to problems associated with our thyroid and digestion. Hydrogenated oils are products such as shortening or margarine. Brominated oils are those put in processed fruit juices to keep them clear.

d. **Water** – drink 1/2 to 2/3 your weight in ounces daily. Distilled water helps to flush toxins out of the body that can lodge in various areas – especially the thyroid. If you use distilled water while cleansing and detoxifying be sure to take a good mineral supplement. When not cleansing, drink good purified water. *See Chapter 3: "Consistently stay hydrated".*

GETTING PROPER NUTRITION

Using the "vegetarian" food guide pyramid, found in Chapter 6: "Develop healthier eating habits", make sure you are eating a balanced diet. We recommend the vegan pyramid for the most benefit, but for those wishing to eat a small portion of eggs or dairy (such as yogurt), following the vegetarian pyramid will still bring health improvements and weight loss.

You need to be consuming plenty of fresh fruits, vegetables and whole grains. Make sure you eat a variety of foods so that you get all of the important nutrients. A deficiency in certain vitamin and minerals can set you up for disease.

To be sure you are getting a variety of foods to complete a balanced diet, be sure you are consuming per day 3 or more servings of vegetables, 5 or more servings of whole grains, 3 or more servings of fruit, 2 or more servings of legumes.

To figure your calorie consumption and fat intake refer to the formulas in Chapter 7: "Incorporate a regular exercise routine". **Try to keep your percentage of fat calories at 20% or less. Remember to never consume less than 1200 calories per day.**

TIPS FOR WEIGHT LOSS

1. Shop after you have eaten, not on an empty stomach. Use a grocery list and stick to it. Avoid prepared foods – get back to basics.

2. Have healthy snacks on hand. Have vegetables cut up and in the refrigerator. Buy low-fat, low-salt and low-sugar crackers, popcorn, etc.

3. Do not keep tempting food in the house. If you do not have it available, chances are you won't even think about it. Keep food stored out of sight. Serve your food from the kitchen so you do not have serving dishes on the table where you are eating.

4. Chew your food thoroughly before swallowing. This will help you to eat slower. Consume less food, it will enhance your digestion and assimilation of nutrients. Avoid watching

T.V or other activities while eating. Focus only on the food and the wonderful benefit it is to your health and well-being.

5. Solicit support from your family. It is very difficult to eat healthy when others around you are eating differently. Even if you do not get the support you want, you will have to be strong. By being an example, your family members may come around as they witness the weight loss and health benefits you are receiving.

6. Educate yourself on nutritional values of foods. Be conscious of the amount of fat and calories you consume each day but do not obsess or stress over it. Once you see the amount and kinds of foods you can consume, you won't have to think about it anymore. You will just be eating healthy.

7. Set reasonable goals that do not seem overwhelming and unobtainable. As an example: Instead of thinking "I have 40 pounds to lose!" think "I will lose 10% of my weight". Maybe that only amounts to 18 pounds (you're at 180 pounds and would like to be at 140 pounds), but it is a reasonable goal. Once you have reached that goal – **reevalua**te. Now you weigh 162 pounds. Maybe you would want to lose another 10% of your weight, but this time it is only 16 pounds. When you reach that goal now, you now weigh 146 pounds. Guess what? Now you only need to lose 6 pounds! Breaking it down like that helps you to focus on obtainable goals that most people can reach.

8. Cook from scratch. It doesn't save much more time cooking from pre-packaged or processed foods.

9. Graze more during the day instead of gorging on fewer meals. Your body will produce less insulin and will store less fat. An example would be to eat 6 small meals

instead of 3 large ones – providing you are consuming the same number of calories.

10. Use vegetarian cookbooks low in fat and sugar. See **I Love to Eat Vegetarian!** cookbook and other "A New Hope for Health" series cookbooks for ideas.

11. Wet saunas are helpful with water retention and in eliminating toxins from our bodies through perspiration. They should be no more than 110 degrees for up to 45 minutes.

12. Colonics and other intestinal cleanses help to eliminate toxins and clean out our colon. They help to improve our digestion and the assimilation of nutrients. We do not feel as hungry or have the desire to snack when our intestines are clean and we are getting plenty of nutrients.

READING NUTRITION LABELS
Learn what the standard definitions are regarding the terms manufactures use on their products.

Milk Lables:

*Fat-free - less than .05 percent, previously labeled as skim milk.
*Low-fat – 1 percent milk
*Reduced-fat – 2 percent milk
Whole – 12 percent fat

Low Calories – 40 calories or less per serving
Calorie-free – less than 5 calories per serving
Light – Either sodium has been reduced 50% or 1/3 less calories or 1/2 the fat
Sugar-free–less than .05 grams.

Fat-free – less than .05 g. of fat per serving.
100% fat-free – same as fat free
Low-fat – 3 g. of fat or less per serving (i.e. 97% fat free)
Reduced –fat – 25% less fat
Low cholesterol – 20mg. or less & 2g. or less saturated fat

HERBAL SUPPLEMENTS THAT MAY HELP

People have use herbal remedies for years and have seen great success. *Check with your health care practitioner regarding your health concerns and which herbs may be the most beneficial.*

Milk thistle – cleanses the liver and helps to stimulate the thyroid.

Cascara sagrada – works as a mild laxative and diuretic.

Dandelion - cleanses the blood, digestive aid, helps to metabolize fat.

Senna – works as a laxative and diuretic

Psyllium – a bulking type of laxative that helps to eliminate waste, helps you to feel full.

Ephedra – helps to stimulate the metabolism and burn fat. Also helps to suppress the appetite. (use this one with caution)

Licorice root – satisfies cravings, helps to balance hormones (too much can cause salt and water retention- do not use for more than one week at a time)

St. John's wort – helps to suppress the appetite and produces a feeling of satiety.

Spirulina – helps to satisfy hunger, rebuilds and purifies the blood, provides needed nutrients and strengthens the body.

Kelp – Norwegian – contains iodine which helps to regulate the thyroid.

Fennel – removes mucous and fat from the intestinal tract, and is an appetite suppressant.

Siberian Ginseng – moves fluids and nutrients throughout the body, reduces stress

Green Tea – improves digestion and helps to metabolize fat.

1.   Write down your food intake for one week.

2.   Compare with the recommended servings on the Food
     Guide Pyramid. Are you consuming a variety of foods?
     Are you consuming enough of each group?

3.   Are you reducing or eliminating your consumption of
     simple carbohydrates (see #1 under Issues to Consider),
     and refined or processed foods (high in calories and fat
     and low in nutrients)?

4.   Using the food guide pyramid, list the foods you/your
     family likes under each of the food groups. Start to build
     your pantry based on the favorite foods. (i.e. corn ,
     whole wheat, oats, fresh and frozen fruits and vegetables
     (avoid canned if possible)

5.   Plan and start a routine, scheduled exercise program.
     Choose activities you enjoy. Remember, aerobic type
     exercises speed up the metabolism and helps to burn
     fat. You must exercise aerobically for at least 20 minutes
     before you start to burn fat. *Chapter 7: "Achieve and
     maintain ideal weight" for more ideas on losing weight.

CHAPTER 9

TRY SAFER, GENTLER APPROACHES TO HEALING AND/OR MAINTAINING ULTIMATE HEALTH

"FIRST, DO NO HARM..."

This is one of the most basic creeds of the medical profession, and originated with Hippocrates when he wrote the oath for physicians to follow, called the Hippocratic Oath. This oath described the patient's rights, physician's responsibilities, and ethical standards in patient care. In many health related fields, graduates are required to recite this oath before licensure or certification. One important point he made was, "As to disease, make a habit of two things – to help, or at least do no harm." Through the years, his words have been reinterpreted into "First, do no harm."

As the medical profession evolved, it has strayed far from this important creed in many ways. Some modern day approaches leave devastating side effects and permanent health problems. There may be times when a drastic or invasive measure is required such as a drug or surgery to save a life, buy a person time to improve his/her health, help an accident victim, or improve the function or appearance of an individual with a birth defect. By using gentler, safer alternative methods either done alone or in conjunction with other therapies, we can improve our overall health, speed up our healing process, and enhance our state of mind.

As with any therapy, what works for one individual

may not work for another. Because there are too many alternative therapies to list in this chapter, I will give a brief description of some that are available to most of us. It is up to each individual to decide which therapy(s) may be most beneficial, accessible, and cost effective. You may need to try different therapies or a combination to gain the most benefit.

There are many gimmicks, products and therapies in the health industry, which claim success. **It is vital that you research any therapy, therapist, or healthcare professional. It is important to use competent, professional, and licensed or certified individuals. Consult your physician or healthcare practitioner before undertaking any treatment.**

ALTERNATIVE THERAPY
AND DIAGNOSIS SYSTEMS

Acupuncture / Acupressure - Acupuncture is a treatment whereby the various acupoints on the meridians of the body are stimulated by inserting tiny acupuncture needles. This therapy helps to improve the flow of energy known as "Chi" or "Qi" through the meridians which helps to restore balance in the body. The insertion of the needles is relatively painless and the treatments are generally relaxing. The acupuncturist can evaluate the health condition by using the pulse or tongue to identify which points should be used. **Acupressure** is similar to acupuncture except generally the fingertips or nails of the therapists are used to apply pressure to the points. The application is less direct than using the needles so the results tend to be a little slower and less specific.

Aromatherapy is the use of the essential oils derived from plants. These oils can be diffused into the air and inhaled, or applied directly to the body. The bottoms of the feet are generally used because the oils can quickly be absorbed into the body via the reflex points. Aromatherapy has been used for thousands of years to help restore health and balance to the body. It has been known to help with conditions such as stress, anxiety, muscular pain, and hormone and digestive problems. Many other conditions have been improved with the use of essential oils.

Chiropractic – uses manipulative techniques and examinations to diagnose and treat disorders associated with muscles, bones, joints, and nerves. It is believed that the spine is the lifeline to the body and keeping it healthy and aligned is the key to good health. People have seen relief from headaches, joint and bone pain, muscle stiffness and spasms, and even asthma and some other internal disorders.

CranioSacral Therapy – non-intrusive, hands-on therapy using a gentle palpation of the cranial sacral bones. Using a light touch, the practitioner uses delicate manual techniques to identify problem areas and then release undo pressure on the brain and spinal cord. CranioSacral Therapy can help alleviate problems such as, headaches, neck and back pain, infantile disorders, traumatic brain and spinal cord injuries, scoliosis, central nervous system disorders, emotional difficulties, learning disabilities, and many other conditions.

Creative Arts Therapy – includes the use of music, dance and movement, and art to improve health and give a sense of well being. They are very beneficial for those with psychological and emotional problems, and physical problems due to stress. Some areas that have been helped are eating conditions, addictions, depression, anxiety, hyperactivity, ADD/ADHD, insomnia, headaches, and digestive problems.

Fasting – is a method of cleansing the body by drinking fluids, eating cleansing foods, or abstaining from solid foods for a specific period of time. Some of the benefits of fasting are: cleanses the body of toxins, speeds up the healing process, boosts the immune system, and gives the digestive system a chance to rest. Many practitioners feel that fasting 1-2 days per month may help prevent serious health problems. Fasting for up to 2 days is considered safe. Fasting for longer than 2 days, or if a person has a serious health problem, is pregnant, or if a small child should be done under supervision of a competent healthcare professional.

Flower and Tree Remedies – are non-toxic extracts from flowers or trees. As with homeopathic remedies, flower/tree remedies are in weak dilutions. They help to balance one physically, mentally, and spiritually. They can also help balance moods and emotions. They can help with negative emotions and personality. Flower and tree remedies can help with conditions such as stress, anxiety, depression, grief, deep-seated mental or emotional problems, nervousness, asthma, skin problems and other chronic health problems such as heart disease and cancer. They can give you an overall sense of well being and calmness.

Galvanic Skin Response Testing (GSR) – GSR is the measurement of the change in the electrical resistance of the skin in response to emotional stimuli. Using electrical signals, it receives feedback from the body in the form of timed GSR measurements. It then analyzes the data giving the practitioner information on general weak and stressed areas of the body. It has helped in areas such as allergies; imbalances in the body; physical, mental and emotional problems; general overall health and wellness.

Guided Imagery – also known as **visualization or thematic imagery**. It is a process of linking the mind to the health problem through meditation and drawing on one's emotional reserves. The person visualizes his/her problem and then visualizes the body's healing process. The theory states that emotions can make us sick as well as make us healthy, and what we think about can become a reality for good or bad. There are books and tapes to help with this process as well as therapists that can teach a person these techniques.

Herbal Medicine – is a therapy involving the use of plants, foods, and nutritional elements to nourish and to heal. Herbs have been used for centuries in most cultures using its local flora and vegetation. Because of the growing concern for the side effects from pharmaceutical drugs, many people are returning to a more natural approach to health, by using herbs and supplements. Herbal remedies have been helpful in treating allergies, arthritis, digestive problems, skin problems, toxic conditions, infections, hormone related problems, arthritis, blood pressure problems, depression, anxiety, and hyperactivity.

Homeopathy – is a medical treatment, which suggests that "like cures like" or The Law of Similars. It uses natural plant, animal, and mineral substances in minute doses of diluted extracts to replicate symptoms of a condition. They induce the body to heal itself. A homeopathic remedy is prescribed based on symptoms and various testing methods. Homeopathic remedies help the body restore balance mentally, emotionally and physically while helping to build the immune system.

Iridology - is a form of assessment suggesting that the iris of the eye is like a map of the human body. It can show weaknesses in various organs, glands, and systems of the body.

An iridologist can recognize the weaknesses in the body and either refer the client to a healthcare practitioner, or help the client devise a plan to improve his/her health. Many iridologists recommend the use herbal supplements, homeopathic remedies, and nutritional supplements to improve the health condition.

Magnetic Therapy – is the use of small magnets attached to the body. They have been reported to help with blood flow and muscles relaxation. Some of the health benefits include reduced joint and muscle pain. They have also helped with tendonitis and bruising.

Massage Therapy – is a therapy that has been providing health benefits for thousands of years. It helps to increase circulation; improve digestion; relax, tone, and strengthen muscles; calm the nervous system; cleanse the lymphatic system; improve tone and elasticity of the skin; reduce the heart rate and lower blood pressure; relieve headaches and insomnia; reduce hyperactivity; increase endorphins which speed up healing and decrease stress by relaxing the mind and body. It can improve the skeletal system by increasing range of motion in the joints and aligning the body. Massage can help to detox the body by helping the elimination system to remove wastes.

Meditation – is an ancient form relaxation and self-healing drawing on our own inner energy. Through deep breathing and focusing of the mind you can lower blood pressure, reduce heart rate, reduce stress and anxiety, bring about calmness, increase mental alertness and concentration. Meditation can improve circulatory problems, headaches, muscular pain, insomnia, respiratory problems, and chronic pain. There are many levels of meditation. There are books and tapes that can help you learn the process, though it is recommended that you have a teacher.

Nutritional Therapy – is using nutrients as food or dietary supplements, and improving the diet to obtain more of the essential nutrients. If deficiency in a nutrient(s) occurs, the environment is ideal for disease and illness. A nutritional therapist may suggest various supplements and diet modifications depending on the specific health concern. Nutritional therapy helps to bring balance and health to the body. It is a great therapy for preventing serious health problems. Nutritional therapy has helped with practically every health problem imaginable.

Osteopathy - is a therapy that works on the skeletal system, the ligaments, muscles and connective tissues of the body through various manipulative techniques. Osteopaths believe that all of our body's systems, including the mind and the emotions, interconnect. If the structural part of our body is out of balance, it can affect any of the other areas of the body. Osteopathy has helped various conditions such as back pain; sciatica; muscle and joint pain; headaches; sinus, digestive, and respiratory problems.

Reflexology – is a therapy whereby the feet, and sometimes the hands, are massaged in a specific way to detect and correct imbalances in the body. Reflexology has been used for thousands of years all over the world. The body is divided into ten equal zones. The foot shows the areas that each zone is connected to. By stimulating the areas on the feet connected to a zone, then other parts of the body on the related zone will be affected. Some conditions which have been helped are: stress, fatigue, hormone imbalances, digestive disturbances, aches and pains, many chronic conditions such as senility, and some common childhood problems.

Reiki – is a Japanese form of healing that taps into the energy that encompasses all living things. The word "Reiki" means "universal life energy". A Reiki practitioner uses his/her hands to direct the flow of healing energies to areas of the body that require healing. Many physical, emotional and spiritual conditions can be improved.

T'ai chi – is an ancient system designed to stimulate and increase "chi" (life energy) in the body. In its flowing, slow movements, it is not only rejuvenating, healing, and relaxing but also a martial art. It is a great daily exercise. T'ai chi has helped conditions such as depression, anxiety, stress, muscle tension, back and joint pain, blood pressure problems, circulatory problems, fatigue and general ill-health.

Yoga – is an ancient form of exercise, meditation, and relaxation that has been around for thousands of years. Yoga postures can help most physical ailments including back problems, arthritis, asthma and other chronic illnesses, stress related disorders, blood pressure problems, circulatory problems, muscle strength and tone, digestive problems, fatigue, insomnia, anxiety and depression.

Zonetherapy (ZoneBalance) – is a treatment using the signals on the feet to identify the areas of weakness, help rejuvenate the cellular system and bring the body and mind into balance. It is more detailed and diagnostic than Reflexology. ZoneBalance improves the structural, endocrine, digestive, excretory, circulatory and central nervous system. It also helps build the immune system, balance the hormones, slow down the aging process, improve the assimilation of nutrients, improve mental function, and prevent disease.

1.   *What are some alternative therapies that would benefit*

me/my family's health the most?

2.   *Which therapy(s) do I have available to me?*

3.   *Which therapy(s) would be the most cost effective?*

4.   *Prioritize the therapies you consider to be the best choice. Remember that you may have to try different therapies or a combination to gain the desired results.*

*Always take the time to research the therapy, the cost of the therapy, the time involved to complete the therapy and the reputation and credentials of the therapist. Referrals are a great place to start.

SUGGESTED WEB SITES AND READING

Listed are various resources available from selected websites and informational books that have been found to be helpful for those wishing to gain more knowledge and understanding on the subjects discussed in this book. Many of these resources contain recipes and ideas for healthy cooking.

WEBSITES
1. www.vegsource.com VegSource
2. www.navigator.tufts.edu Tufts Nutrition Navigator
3. www.drweil.com Dr. Weil Homepage
4. www.altmedicine.com Alternative Medicine
5. www.holisticmedicine.org American Holistic Medical Association
6. www.vetetariantimes.com Vegetarian Times Magazine
7. www.betternutrition.com Better Nutrition Magazine

BOOKS
1. Schmidt, M., Smith, L. H., Sehnert, W.K., *Beyond Antibiotics,* North Atlantic Books, Berkeley, CA, 1993.
2. Clark, H., *The Cure for All Disease,* New Century Press, San Diego, CA, 1995.
3. Lipski, E. *Digestive Wellness,*Keats, Publishing, Inc., New Canaan, CN, 1996.
4. Cheraskin,E., Ringdorf, W.M. Jr., Clark, J.W., *Diet and Disease,* Keats, Publishing, Inc., New Canaan, CN, 1995.
5. Blaylock, R. L., *EXCITOTOXINS-The Taste That Kills,* Health Press, Santa Fe, NM, 1997.
6. Erasmus, U., *Fats that Heal, Fats that Kill,* Alive Books, Burnaby BC Canada, 1993.
7. Diamond, H., *Fit For Life,* Warner Books, New York, NY,

1985
8. Colbin, A., *Food and Healing,* Ballantine Books, New York, 1996.
9. Pitchford, P., *Healing With Whole Foods,* North Atlantic Books, Berkeley, CA, 1993
10. Page, L., *Healthy Healing,* Healthy Healing Publications, 1998.
11. Weil, A. *Health and Healing,* Houghton Mifflin Company, Boston, NY, 1998.
12. Sorenson, M. *Mega Health,* National Institute of Fitness, Ivins, UT, 1993.
13. Balch, P., *Prescription for Nutritional Healing,* Avery Books, NY, 2000
14. Hoffer, A., Morton, W. *Smart Nutrients,* Avery Publishing Group, Garden City Park, NY, 1994.
15. Jensen, B., *Tissue Cleansing Through Bowel Management,* Escondido, CA, 1981.
16. Klaper, M., *Vegan Nutrition: Pure and Simple,* Gentle World, Inc. Paia, Maui, HI, 1997.
17. Batmanghelidj, B., *Your Body's Many Cries for Water, Global Health Solutions, Inc,* Falls Church, VA, 1997.

MAGAZINES
1. Vegetarian Times
2. Veggie Life
3. Organic Gardening. Rodale Inc.1998
4. Better Nutrition-free in local health food stores
5. Prevention

INDEX